Musculoskeletal System

Anil H. Walji, MD, PhD

Professor and Director, Division of Anatomy
Professor of Radiology and Diagnostic Imaging
Professor of Surgery
Faculty of Medicine and Dentistry
University of Alberta
Edmonton, Alberta, Canada

UK edition authors
Sîan Knight, Sona V. Biswas, and Rehana Iqbal

UK series editor
Daniel Horton-Szar

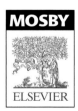

MOSBY

ELSEVIER

1600 John F. Kennedy Boulevard
Suite 1800
Philadelphia, PA 19103-2899

CRASH COURSE: MUSCULOSKELETAL SYSTEM   ISBN-13: 978-1-4160-3008-9
Copyright © 2006 by Mosby, Inc., an affiliate of Elsevier Inc.   ISBN-10: 1-4160-3008-5

Adapted from Crash Course Muscles, Bones and Skin 2e by Sîan Knight, ISBN 0-7234-3291-0. © 2003, Elsevier Science Limited. All rights reserved.

The rights of Sîan Knight to be identified as the author of this work have been asserted by her in accordance with the Copyright Designs and Patents Act, 1988.

Library of Congress Cataloging-in-Publication Data

Walji, Anil H.
    Crash Course: musculoskeletal system/Anil H. Walji.—1st American ed.
        p. ; cm.—(Crash course)
    Includes index.
    ISBN 1-4160-3008-5
    1. Musculoskeletal system—Physiology—Outlines, syllabi, etc.   2. Musculoskeletal system—Diseases—Diagnosis—Outlines, syllabi, etc.   3. Skin—Physiology—Outlines, syllabi etc.
    4. Skin—Diseases—Diagnosis—Outlines, syllabi, etc.   I. Title: Musculoskeletal system.
    II. Title.   III. Series.
    [DNLM: 1. Musculoskeletal System.   2. Musculoskeletal Diseases.   3. Musculoskeletal Physiology.   4. Skin Diseases.   5. Skin Physiology. WE 100 W176c 2006]
    QP301.W274 2006
    612.7—dc22   2005056106

Commissioning Editor: Alex Stibbe
Developmental Editor: Stan Ward
Project Manager: David Saltzberg
Design: Andy Chapman
Cover Design: Antbits Illustration
Illustration Manager: Mick Ruddy

Printed in China.

Last digit is the print number:
9 8 7 6 5 4 3 2 1

CRASH COURSE

Musculoskeletal System

Other Titles in ... Course Series

There are 23 books in the Crash Cou... ...es in two ranges: Basic Science and Clinical. Each book follows the same format, with concise text, clear illustrations, and helpful learning features, including access online USMLE test questions.

Basic Science titles
Pathology
Nervous System
Renal and Urinary Systems
Gastrointestinal System
Respiratory System
Endocrine and Reproductive Systems
Metabolism and Nutrition
Pharmacology
Immunology
Musculoskeletal System
Cardiovascular System

Forthcoming:
Cell Biology and Genetics
Anatomy

Clinical titles
Surgery
Cardiology
History and Examination
Internal Medicine
Neurology
Gastroenterology

Forthcoming:
OBGYN
Psychiatry
Imaging
Pediatrics

Preface

Crash Course: Musculoskeletal System provides a comprehensive yet concise overview of the structure and function of the musculoskeletal system and skin in health and disease. The book is divided into three main sections. The first section deals with the basic structure and function of muscles, bones, joints, and skin; the second covers the clinical aspects of rheumatology, orthopedics, and dermatology; and the third, intended to familiarize the reader with board type examination questions, is on self-assessment.

The format of this book is designed primarily to meet the needs of students and residents who have limited time to learn huge amounts of material to pass examinations and become competent physicians, which is the majority of us! Having been there and done that, I can assure you that you will find this book a most refreshing strategy for mastering a large and complex body of basic and clinical information relatively painlessly.

The approach used by the authors in creating this compact, user-friendly text is particularly suitable for students who have studied medicine within an integrated, systems-based curriculum with an emphasis on communication skills, problem solving, and self-directed learning. Students and residents from more traditional curricula will also find this book a useful tool for reviewing the subject quickly and efficiently.

The text is presented in compact, fully integrated, easy-to-manage sections with emphasis on clinical correlation throughout to facilitate comprehension and reduce the fear of learning facts. A new and expanded section on history and physical examination gives practical advice on improving communication skills and interactions with the patient. I hope you find *Crash Course: Musculoskeletal System* a useful tool in helping you to master this information, and I wish you success in your examinations and in your careers.

Anil H. Walji, MD, PhD

Acknowledgments

I would like to acknowledge and thank my wife, Parviz, for her patience with me and for her constant support, encouragement, and nurturing love, without which I could not possibly have accomplished this, nor any of my numerous other tasks. I would also like to thank my "kids," Farah and Amreen, for keeping me modest, honest, and firmly planted on the ground and for opening my eyes to so many other perspectives that life has to offer. My sincere gratitude also goes to Alex Stibbe, Rachel Wheeler, Trevor MacDougall, Stan Ward, Laura Mason, David Saltzberg, and all the wonderful people at Elsevier for their patience and for their constant guidance, support, and encouragement throughout this project. Finally, I would like to gratefully acknowledge all my colleagues who have supported me through this endeavor.

Plates 1–24 are from White G: Levene's Color Atlas of Dermatology, 2nd ed. St. Louis, Mosby, 1997.

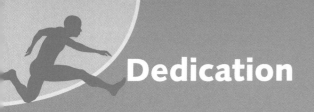

Dedication

*To
my wife and two daughters,
without whom I would not be who
or where I am today.*

Contents

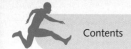

BASIC MEDICAL SCIENCE OF MUSCLES, BONES, AND SKIN

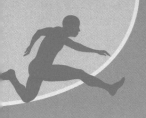

1. Musculoskeletal System: An Overview

The musculoskeletal system comprises muscles, bones, and joints. It makes up most of the body's mass and performs several essential functions, including:

- The maintenance of body shape.
- The support and protection of soft tissue structures.
- Movement.
- Breathing.
- The storage of calcium and phosphate in bone.

Connective tissue

Most of the musculoskeletal system is made up of connective tissue such as bone and cartilage. Connective tissue comprises specialized cells embedded in an extracellular matrix of collagen, elastin, and structural proteoglycans. In bone, this matrix is mineralized and rigid.

Muscle

There are three types of muscle: skeletal, cardiac, and smooth (Fig. 1.1).

- Skeletal muscle is striated muscle controlled by the somatic nervous system. Most muscle in the body is of this type.
- Cardiac muscle is striated muscle of the heart controlled by the autonomic nervous system.
- Smooth muscle is nonstriated muscle controlled by a variety of chemical mediators and the autonomic nervous system. Smooth muscle is important in the function of most tissues (e.g., blood vessels, the gastrointestinal and reproductive tracts).

Energy is stored in tissues as adenosine triphosphate (ATP) and is converted by muscle tissue into mechanical energy. This produces movement or tension. The contraction of muscle

Properties of the three different muscle types			
	Skeletal	**Cardiac**	**Smooth**
Histologic appearance	Cross-striated, multinucleated muscle fibers	Cross-striated, single nucleated muscle fibers containing intercalated discs	Nonstriated, spindle cells with a single nucleus
Site	Skeletal covering	Muscular component of the heart	Found in wall of blood vessel, airways glands, and walls of hollow organs
Cell size	50–60 μm in diameter, up to 10 cm long	15 μm in diameter, 100 μm long	2–10 μm in diameter, 20–400 μm long
Control	Voluntary/reflex; controlled by somatic nervous sytem	Self-regulated by pacemaker cells; heart rate can be altered by autonomic nervous system	Involuntary control or regulation by inherent contraction initiation (visceral smooth muscle)
Nature of contraction	Rapid contraction and relaxation	Spontaneous and rhythmic contraction	Slow and sustained contraction
Function	Voluntary movement of skeleton and posture maintenance	Contractions pump blood around the body	Related to the structure, (e.g., regulation of blood vessel diameter, hair erection)

Fig. 1.1 Properties of the three different types of muscle.

requires stimulation. The type of stimulation varies; for example, skeletal muscle is activated by motor neurons, cardiac muscle initiates its own contractions (which are regulated by the autonomic nervous system), and smooth muscle is activated by a variety of chemical mediators and the autonomic nervous system. Stimulation of muscle causes protein filaments in its cells, called actin and myosin, to interact and thus produce a contractile force.

The skeleton

The skeleton consists of bone, cartilage, and fibrous ligaments. A joint is the site where bones are united with each other by fibrous capsules and ligaments. The range of movement at the joint and the rigidity or flexibility of a joint depend on how the bones articulate together.

Bone
Bone is rigid and forms most of the skeleton. It functions as a supportive framework for the musculoskeletal system, and the bony sites for muscle attachment provide the mechanical basis for locomotion. Other functions of bone include mineral storage in its matrix and formation of blood cells (hematopoiesis) in the marrow.

Cartilage
Cartilage is a resilient tissue that provides semirigid support in some parts of the skeleton. Cartilage is also a component of some joint types. Most bone is formed in a cartilaginous template during development.

Ligaments, tendons, and aponeuroses
Ligaments, tendons, and aponeuroses are fibrous tissues that connect the various components of the musculoskeletal system.
- Ligaments are flexible but strong bands that connect bones or cartilage together, strengthening and stabilizing joints.
- Tendons are connections between muscle and bone.
- An aponeurosis may be considered as a broad, sheet-like tendon.

Joints
Joints are composite structures between bones. They may also include cartilage and fibrous connective tissue. There are several types of joint. The strength of a joint and the range of movement it allows depend on its position and function.

Control of the musculoskeletal system
The musculoskeletal system is controlled by the somatic nervous system to produce coordinated movements and locomotion. A number of elements contribute to the somatic nervous system's control:
- Efferent motor neurons activate groups of muscle fibers to produce a contraction.
- Afferent feedback from stretch receptors in muscles and tendons and from sensory nerve endings in joints and skin allows coordination of movement.
- Neural pathways in the spinal cord coordinate the action of related muscle groups (e.g., agonist/antagonist pairs) and also initiate repetitive actions, such as walking ("central pattern generator").

For more information about central control of movement and locomotion, refer to *Crash Course: Nervous System, 2nd ed.*

Skin

Structure
The skin is composed of three layers: an outer protective epidermis, an inner connective tissue dermis, and a fatty subcutaneous layer (Fig. 1.2). It is characterized by a tough keratinized surface that protects underlying tissues from the external environment. The epidermis is designed essentially for withstanding abrasive forces and wear and tear.

The thickness of skin varies depending on its location on the body. The epidermis is usually around 0.1 mm thick; however, this thickness increases to between 0.8 and 1.4 mm in places, such as in the soles of the feet and the palms of the hands where it undergoes repeated trauma. The dermis follows this pattern, ranging from 0.6 mm thickness on the eyelids to 3 mm on the palms and soles. The subcutaneous layer (subcutis, superficial fascia) of the skin is much thicker than the layers above and has a different thickness distribution: it is thickest on the abdomen, where it may reach depths of 3 cm or more.

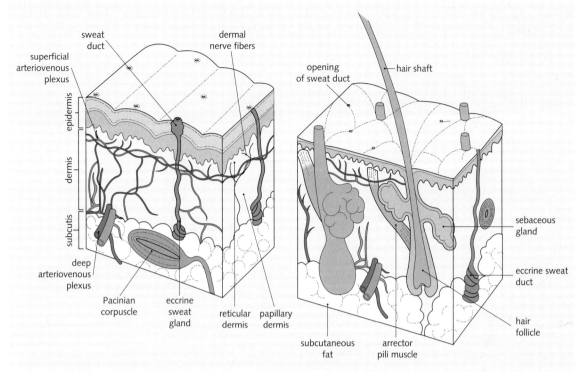

Fig. 1.2 The structure of the skin (adapted from *Dermatology: An Illustrated Colour Text*, 2nd ed., by Gawkrodger DJ, Churchill Livingstone, 1997).

Functions

The skin performs many functions in addition to its main protective role. These functions include thermoregulation; synthesis of vitamin D and various hormones; and the perception of pain, temperature, and touch sensations.

Skin derivatives

There are many derivatives of skin, including hair, nails, sebaceous glands, and sweat glands, which will also be discussed in this book. These structures are so named because they have developed from cells derived from the epidermis. They perform important functions in both the protection and homeostasis of the skin.

Pathology

Because of the skin's exposure to the external environment, it is open to insults caused by infection and infestation. This subject, as well as the clinical manifestations caused by the usual gamut of pathology (e.g., inflammation, tumors, genetic disorders, systemic disease, and drug-induced disorders), will be covered in Chapter 8.

Connective tissue

Definition

Connective tissue is a basic type of tissue. It contains cells embedded in an extracellular matrix of ground substance and fibers. Connective tissue is characterized by a high matrix:cell ratio.

Origins

Connective tissue is derived from the embryonic mesoderm and neural crest. These differentiate into the embryonic connective tissue or mesenchyme (Fig. 1.3).

Functions

Connective tissue performs several functions. These include:

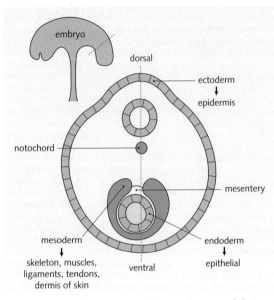

Fig. 1.3 The three primitive embryonic layers and their derivative structures.

- Mediating the exchange of nutrients and metabolic products between tissues and the circulatory system.
- Providing mechanical support (physical) as well as allowing for muscle attachment.
- Packaging, because connective tissue encloses and lies between other specialized tissues.
- Performing a metabolic role and allowing fat storage in adipose tissue.
- Providing insulation.
- Allowing for defense and repair, with some cells involved in the immune response.

Classification and components

Connective tissue is classified according to its function, location, structure, and properties (Fig. 1.4). The three main components of connective tissue are cells, fibers, and ground substance.

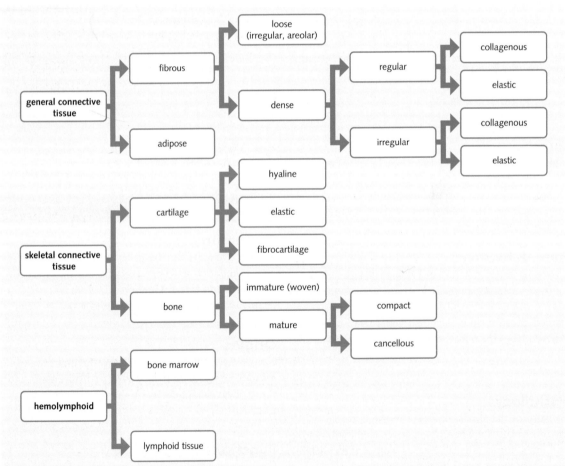

Fig. 1.4 Classification of connective tissue.

Cells

Connective tissue comprises several cell types. Each of these cell types performs a certain function (Fig. 1.5).

Fibers
Collagen

Collagen is the main fiber found in the extracellular matrix of connective tissue. Collagen is produced from tropocollagen, a substance synthesized by the endoplasmic reticulum of matrix-secreting cells.

Connective tissue cell types and functions		
	Cell type	Functions
Fixed cells	Fibroblasts, chondroblasts, osteoblasts, osteoclasts	Synthesis and maintenance of matrix
	Adipocytes	Fat metabolism
	Mast cells	Release of histamine
	Mesenchymal cells	Mature cell precursors
Transient cells	White blood cells	Defense and immune response
	Melanocytes	Pigmentation

Fig. 1.5 Connective tissue cell types and their functions.

Tropocollagen becomes modified to collagen when it is released into the extracellular matrix.

Collagen contains three helical polypeptide chains (Fig. 1.6). Differences in these chains result in at least 15 types of collagen molecules, each with a particular function (Fig. 1.7).

Elastin

Elastin is a component of elastic fibers. Elastic fibers are found in the skin, elastic cartilage, fibrous joint capsules, ligaments, lungs, and blood vessels. They are thinner than collagen and are arranged in random networks in irregular connective tissue and in parallel bundles in elastic ligaments. In the larger arteries, elastic fibers are arranged in the arterial wall in concentric circles.

Elastin is produced from proelastin, a substance synthesized by matrix-secreting cells. Proelastin is modified to elastin by the cell's Golgi apparatus when it is released into the extracellular matrix.

Structural proteoglycans

Structural proteoglycans provide a ground substance surrounding the cells and fibers of connective tissue. They contain protein chains bound to branched polysaccharides and form fibers such as fibronectin and laminin. Some structural proteoglycans are

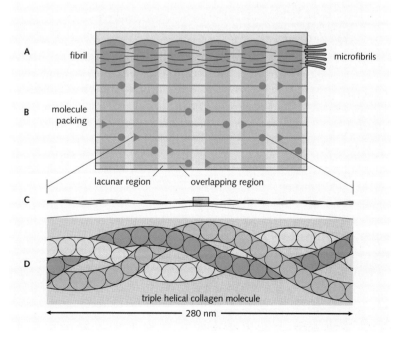

Fig. 1.6 Microstructure of the collagen fibril. A. Microfibril. B. Packing of molecules. C. Collagen molecule. D. Triple helix of polypeptide (α) chains.

Functions of collagen types		
Type	Location	Function
I	Skin, tendon, ligaments, bone, fascia, and organ capsules (accounts for 90% of body collagen)	Provides variable mechanical support (loose or dense)
II	Hyaline and elastic cartilage, notochord, and intervertebral discs	Provides shape and resistance to pressure
III	Connective tissue of organs (liver, lymphoid organs), blood vessels, and fetal skin	Forms reticular networks
IV	Basement membrane of epithelial and endothelial cells	Provides support and a filtration barrier
V	Basement membrane of smooth and skeletal muscle cells	Provides support (other functions poorly understood)

Fig. 1.7 Functions of the different types of collagen.

found on the surface of cells, and here their functions include cell-to-cell recognition, adhesion, and migration.

Communication between cells and their environment is facilitated by the structural proteoglycans that function as cell adhesion molecules (CAMs). In doing so, the proteoglycans regulate a large number of cell functions, including proliferation, gene expression, apoptosis, and differentiation. In the future, modifying the actions of adhesion molecules may be the key to treating illnesses such as cancer.

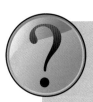

- List the components of the musculoskeletal system.
- Describe the general functions of the musculoskeletal system.
- Describe the mechanisms, stimulation, and regulation of skeletal, cardiac, and smooth muscle types.
- List the general functions of the skin.
- Name the three layers of the skin.
- Define connective tissue.
- List the functions of connective tissue.
- Give a simple classification of connective tissue.

2. Skeletal Muscle

Comparison of the three muscle types

Muscle is a tissue made up of contractile cells. These cells are capable of producing movement or tension. Other examples of contractile cells include myoepithelial cells and myofibroblasts that are found in connective tissue.

Three types of muscle tissue are found in the human body: skeletal, cardiac, and smooth (Fig. 2.1). Cardiac and smooth muscle types are discussed in more detail in Chapter 3.

Skeletal muscle
The alternative names for skeletal muscle are striated (from its histologic appearance) or voluntary (from the mechanism by which contraction is controlled).

Sites
The majority of muscle found in the body is skeletal (Fig. 2.2). Skeletal muscle is found in the head and neck, face, limbs, thorax, abdominal wall, and pelvis.

Control
Contraction of skeletal muscle is generally voluntary, but it may also occur as a reflex (e.g., withdrawing rapidly from a harmful stimulus). Contraction is controlled by the somatic nervous system.

Histologic appearance
Skeletal muscle cells are long and thin and are therefore often referred to as muscle fibers. The cells are multinucleated and appear cross-striated under light microscopy.

Cell size
Skeletal muscle cells are 50–60 μm in diameter (range 10–100 μm) and up to 10 cm long.

Nature of contraction
Rapid contraction and relaxation of skeletal muscle occurs as a twitch. The nature of the stimulus is important because contractions may summate to produce smooth and sustained contractions if the muscle is stimulated rapidly and repetitively.

Function
Skeletal muscle has an important role in voluntary movement of the skeleton and maintenance of posture. It is also involved in the movement of the tongue and the eyeball in the orbit.

Cardiac muscle
Cardiac muscle is found in the myocardium, the middle layer of the heart. These cells are also referred to as myocardial fibers.

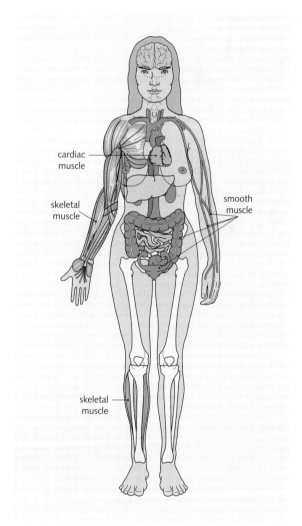

Fig. 2.1 Location of the different muscle types in the human body.

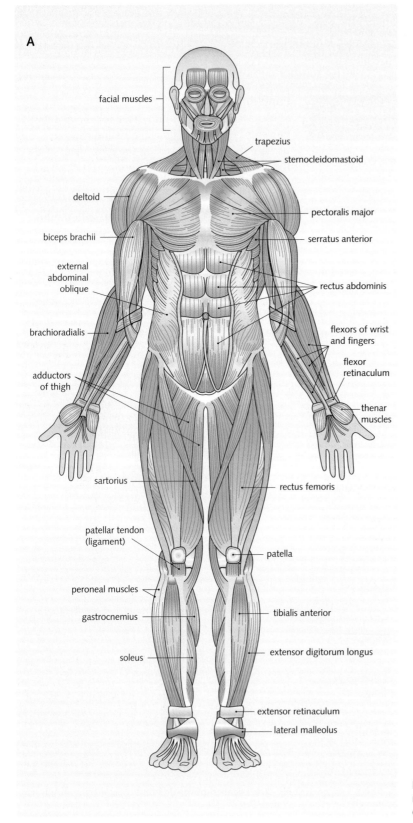

A

facial muscles

trapezius

sternocleidomastoid

deltoid

pectoralis major

biceps brachii

serratus anterior

external
abdominal
oblique

rectus abdominis

brachioradialis

flexors of wrist
and fingers

flexor
retinaculum

adductors
of thigh

thenar
muscles

sartorius

rectus femoris

patellar tendon
(ligament)

patella

peroneal muscles

gastrocnemius

tibialis anterior

soleus

extensor digitorum longus

extensor retinaculum

lateral malleolus

Fig. 2.2 A. Anterior view of major
muscle groups in the body (courtesy
of Dr. KM Backhouse).

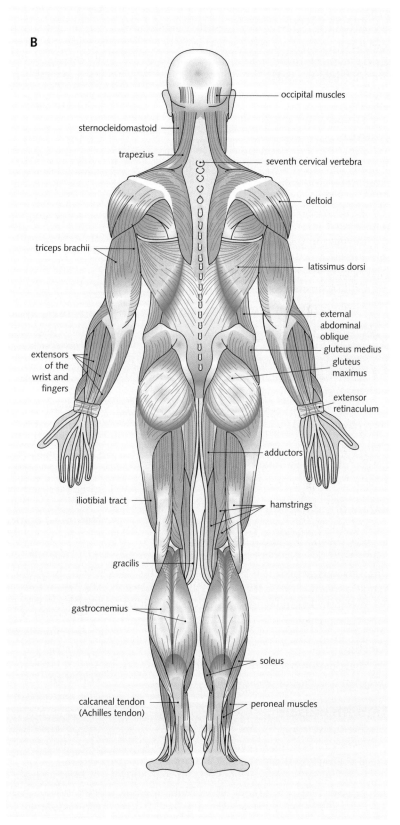

Fig. 2.2 B. Posterior view of major muscle groups in the body (courtesy of Dr. KM Backhouse).

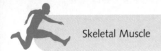

Sites

The myocardium forms the muscular component of the heart (see Fig. 2.1) and lies between the pericardium externally and the endocardium internally (see Fig. 3.1).

Control

Contraction of the myocardium is regulated by pacemaker cells in the tissue. The autonomic nervous system can modify contraction of myocardium by the duration and strength of contraction, therefore altering the heart rate.

Histologic appearance

With cardiac muscle, as with skeletal muscle, longitudinal and transverse striations are seen under light microscopy. However, cardiac muscle cells are smaller and branched and have single, central nuclei. Intercellular junctions are often seen and are called intercalated discs.

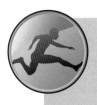

Cardiac muscle is a type of striated muscle, and its properties can be considered to lie between those of smooth and skeletal muscle types.

Cell size

Cardiac muscle cells (myocardial fibers) are 15 μm in diameter and 100 μm in length.

Nature of contraction

Cardiac muscle cells within the myocardium undergo spontaneous and rhythmic contractions. These contractions are always brief twitches followed by a long refractory period. This period enables cardiac muscle to relax, allowing the heart to fill with blood. Because of the long refractory period after each brief twitch, summation of contractions does not occur.

Function

The myocardium pumps deoxygenated blood to the lungs and oxygenated blood to the body tissues.

Smooth muscle

The alternative name for smooth muscle is involuntary muscle, named after the mechanism by which contraction is controlled.

Smooth muscle can be divided into visceral (single unit or syncytial) or multiunit types. Most smooth muscle is of the visceral type.

Sites

Single-unit smooth muscle is found in small blood vessels, the ducts of secretory glands, and the walls of hollow organs of the gastrointestinal and urogenital systems (see Fig. 2.1). Multiunit smooth muscle is found in large blood vessels, large airways, the eyes, and hair follicles.

Control

Smooth muscle contraction is always under involuntary control. In the case of visceral smooth muscle, initiation of contraction is inherent (caused by pacemaker cells in the smooth muscle tissue that discharge in an irregular pattern) and can be modified by hormones, local metabolites, and the autonomic nervous system. Multiunit smooth muscle, however, is neurogenic (the initiation of each contraction is under the control of the autonomic nervous system).

Histologic appearance

Smooth muscle is less organized than skeletal muscle and myocardium, and no striations are seen under light microscopy. The cells are spindle-shaped and have large, single, central nuclei.

Cell size

Smooth muscle cells are 2–10 μm in diameter and 20–400 μm long. Cell size varies, depending on location; for example, cells of 20 μm are found in small blood vessels, while cells up to 400 μm in length are found in the uterus.

Nature of contraction

Low-force contraction of smooth muscle occurs with relatively little energy expenditure. In the case of multiunit smooth muscle, individual muscle fibers contract via the same mechanism as in skeletal muscle. In visceral smooth muscle, however, the whole muscle mass contracts and not individual muscle fibers, meaning that contraction is slow and sustained.

Function

The functions of smooth muscle are related to the structure in which they are found; for example, the smooth muscle component of blood vessels regulates blood flow by altering the diameter of the blood vessels.

Multiunit smooth muscle is involved in the alteration of pupil size by contraction of muscles in the iris, and it is involved in accommodation by contraction of the ciliary muscle. Multiunit smooth muscle is also responsible for "goose bumps," which result from contraction of muscle at the base of each hair follicle.

Skeletal and multiunit smooth muscle types may be referred to as neurogenic muscle (i.e., muscle in which contraction arises as a result of nerve stimulation).

Cardiac and visceral smooth muscle types may be referred to as myogenic muscle (i.e., they require no nerve stimulation for contraction that arises from within the muscle, owing to the presence of pacemaker cells).

Skeletal muscle

The contraction generated by a muscle depends on:
- The length of the muscle fibers.
- The volume/number of muscle fibers.
- The rate at which fiber length changes.

The range of movement produced by a muscle is proportional to the length of the muscle fibers; however, the bulkier the muscle, the greater the force it will generate. This can be illustrated by the following example. Consider two pieces of muscle tissue that are of equal volume. One is long and narrow, and the other is short but broad in cross-section. The long muscle will allow a greater degree of shortening, but it cannot generate much contraction force because of its narrow cross-section. By contrast, the shorter muscle cannot contract over any great length, but it generates a large contraction force because its cross-section incorporates many muscle fibers.

Muscles assume a variety of shapes, depending on the type of contraction involved. For example, a multipennate arrangement results in a large number of short fibers attached to a single tendon, and the force of contraction is great and concentrated on the tendon (Fig. 2.3).

Muscle groups are arranged in pairs that consist of:
- A functional group in which one muscle is the main participant and the other muscles help to perform a movement. For example, flexion at the elbow joint is due to the action of biceps with the help of brachialis, brachioradialis, and the forearm flexor muscles.
- An antagonistic group in which muscles oppose the movement of the functional group. For example, the triceps, assisted by the anconeus, antagonize the action of biceps by causing extension at the elbow (Fig. 2.4).

A muscle can belong to more than one group. For example, the latissimus dorsi is involved in both adduction and extension of the shoulder joint.

Each end of a muscle is usually attached to bone. The origin, or head, is the attachment site at which there is little movement when the muscle performs its main action (Fig. 2.5). The insertion is the more mobile attachment site.

The terms proximal and distal attachment may be more appropriate because, depending on movement, the origin (proximal attachment) may be more mobile than the insertion (distal attachment).

Muscles are attached to bone by fibrous connective tissue, although not all skeletal muscle is attached to bone (e.g., some muscles controlling facial expression). The muscles of the tongue, however, are attached to the mandible, styloid process of the skull, and the hyoid bone. In addition, rings of skeletal muscle or sphincters (e.g., the external urethral sphincter that controls passage of urine from the bladder to the urethra) do not attach to bone. Other structures associated with skeletal muscle are presented in the following paragraphs.

Tendons
A tendon is an inelastic, flexible cord consisting of closely packed collagen fibers. The tendon attaches muscle to bone and possesses immense tensile strength.

Aponeuroses
An aponeurosis is a thin, broad sheet of fibrous connective tissue attaching muscle to bone. It is found in muscles that have a wide attachment area to bone (e.g., the anterior abdominal wall). An aponeurotic sheet is, in essence, a broad tendon.

Sesamoid bones
A sesamoid bone is a small bone found in the tendons of certain muscles (e.g., the patella and some bones in the hand and foot). Its presence may correlate with sites susceptible to wear and tear. The bone may also provide extra leverage.

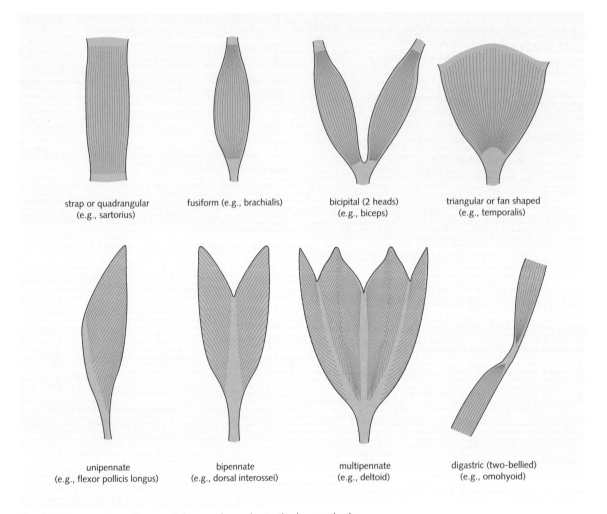

strap or quadrangular
(e.g., sartorius)

fusiform (e.g., brachialis)

bicipital (2 heads)
(e.g., biceps)

triangular or fan shaped
(e.g., temporalis)

unipennate
(e.g., flexor pollicis longus)

bipennate
(e.g., dorsal interossei)

multipennate
(e.g., deltoid)

digastric (two-bellied)
(e.g., omohyoid)

Fig. 2.3 Fiber configurations and shapes of muscles in the human body.

Microstructure of skeletal muscle
Arrangement of muscle tissue

Whole muscle consists of fibers that are arranged in bundles called fasciculi. Connective tissue lies between the individual muscle fibers and fasciculi; in addition, a dense connective tissue coat surrounds the whole muscle (see Fig. 2.5).

Skeletal muscle has a rich blood supply. The blood vessels and nerves divide and extend throughout the perimysium (the collagen connective tissue that surrounds fasciculi). Smaller fasciculi are found in muscles involved in fine movement; hence, the size of fasciculi is suggestive of function.

Microenvironment of skeletal muscle

Skeletal muscle fibers are arranged in parallel in a fasciculus (Fig. 2.6). Although skeletal muscle fibers are long, they do not extend the whole length of the muscle but are organized as overlapping bundles. This arrangement enables the force of a contraction to be transmitted throughout the muscle.

Skeletal muscle fibers can be divided into three types: I, IIa, and IIb. All three types are widely distributed throughout the muscle (Fig. 2.7). The properties of the different types of muscle fibers are considered in more detail on p. 31.

Sarcomere

Muscle fibers, or myofibers, are cells containing myofibrils. Myofibrils consist of myofilaments arranged in contractile units called sarcomeres. Two types of myofilaments occur:

- Thick filaments, mainly composed of myosin protein.
- Thin filaments, mainly composed of actin protein.

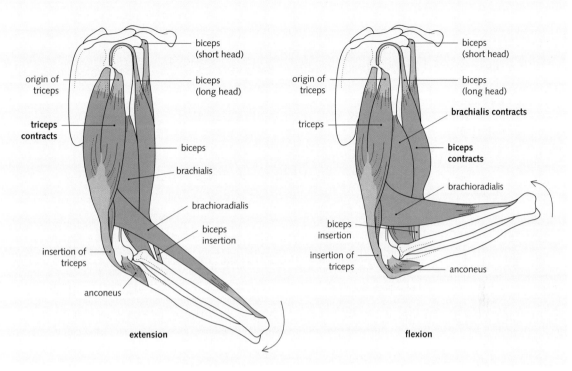

Fig. 2.4 Arrangement of muscles in antagonistic pairs demonstrated at the elbow joint.

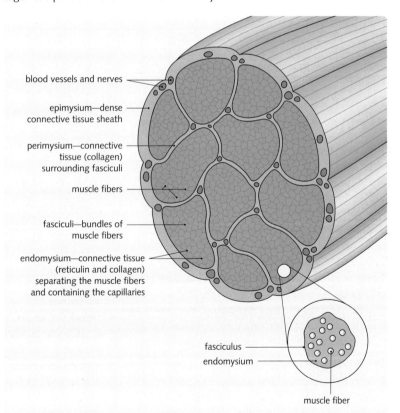

Fig. 2.5 Cross-section of whole muscle showing the arrangement of muscles into fasciculi and fibers surrounded by connective tissue.

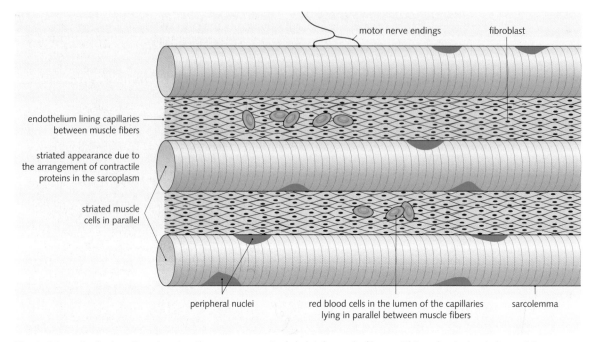

Fig. 2.6 Longitudinal section showing the arrangement of skeletal muscle fibers within a fasciculus (schematic).

Classification of different types of skeletal muscle fibers			
Fiber type	Color	Speed and force of twitch	Resistance to fatigue
I	Red (because of myoglobin)	Slow, only 10% of force of type IIb	High (fatigue resistant)
IIa	Intermediate	Fast, but force and speed less than type IIb	Intermediate (fatigue resistant)
IIb	White	Fast and high force	Low (fatigue after repeated stimulation), fast, fatigable

Fig. 2.7 Classification of the different types of skeletal muscle fibers.

The organization of these myofilaments leads to the striated appearance of skeletal muscle (Figs. 2.8 and 2.9).

Cellular structure of muscle fiber

A muscle fiber is a specialized cell (Fig. 2.10) that comprises:
- A sarcolemma or cell membrane.
- Sarcoplasm or cytoplasm.
- A sarcoplasmic reticulum or endoplasmic reticulum.

Each muscle fiber cell has multiple peripheral nuclei, glycogen granules, and mitochondria that lie in the sarcoplasm between myofibrils. They contain T tubules—channels that extend from the sarcolemma of the muscle fiber and surround each muscle fiber at the junction of the A and I band, called the AI junction. T tubules ensure that all sarcomere contractions are synchronized.

Sarcoplasmic reticulum runs longitudinally along myofibrils and wraps around groups of myofibrils. In regions of T tubules, the sarcoplasmic reticulum forms terminal cisternae.

Within the muscle, the triad is an important structure that consists of a T tubule with sarcoplasmic reticulum on either side. Depolarization is transmitted through the T tubule, causing release of Ca^{2+} into the sarcoplasm and triggering muscular contraction.

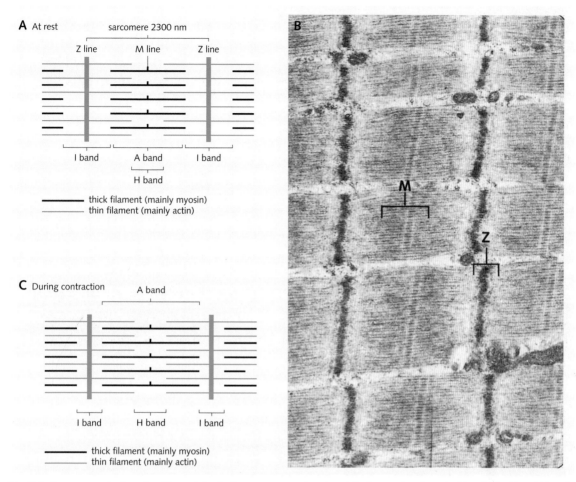

Fig. 2.8 Arrangement of contractile proteins in the sarcomere at rest and during contraction. A. At rest, the H and I bands represent areas in which the thick and thin filaments do not overlap. The Z line anchors the actin filaments, and the M line anchors the myosin filaments. B. The pattern of actin and myosin filaments is demonstrated clearly on the electron micrograph. C. During contraction, the Z lines "slide" closer together, causing shortening of muscle. The A band remains constant in width, but the I and H bands shorten (M, M line; Z, Z line) (electron micrograph courtesy of Dr. T Gray).

Replacement of muscle fibers

Satellite cells are small, spindle-shaped cells that lie between the sarcolemma and basal lamina in adult skeletal muscle; they are visible under electron microscopy. If muscle damage occurs but the basal lamina remains intact, several events occur:

- Satellite cells proliferate to form myoblasts.
- Myoblasts fuse to form myotubules around which myofibrils assemble.
- New muscle fibers form in which the nuclei are centrally rather than peripherally placed.

If the basal lamina becomes damaged, fibroblasts are activated to repair the tissues, with resulting scar formation.

Cellular physiology of skeletal muscle

Ion balance and the resting membrane potential

There are differences in the ionic composition of the intracellular fluid (ICF) and extracellular fluid (ECF) of muscle cells (Fig. 2.11). These differences are due to:

- The selective permeability of the cell membrane to K^+ and Cl^-.
- The presence of large intracellular impermeable anions from amino acid metabolism. These cause

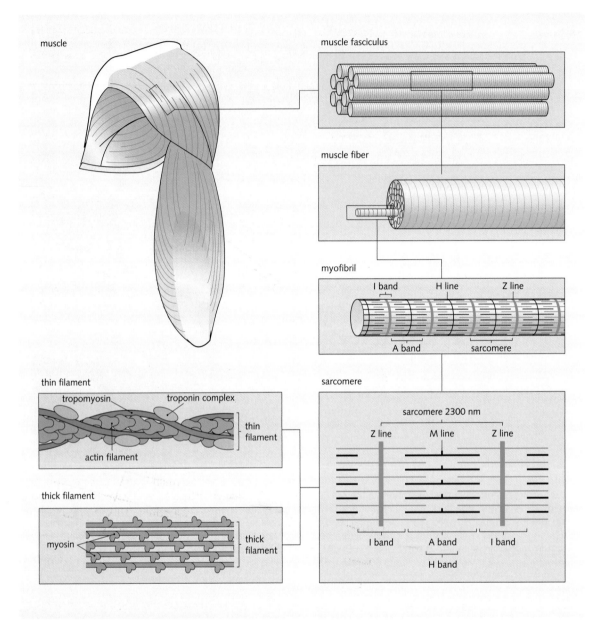

Fig. 2.9 Organization of skeletal muscle.

movement of Cl^- extracellularly and K^+ intracellularly.
• Relative cell membrane impermeability to Na^+.

Resting membrane potential
The resting membrane potential (RMP) is the difference in voltage between the inside and the outside of the cell at rest, normally a value of −90 mV in muscle cells. This separation of charge across the cell membrane creates the potential to do work and is a result of the differences in the distribution and permeabilities of ions across the cell membrane (Fig. 2.12).

The movement of ions across the cell membrane that causes the voltage difference is caused by:
• A concentration gradient that favors K^+ efflux.
• An electrostatic gradient that favors K^+ influx.

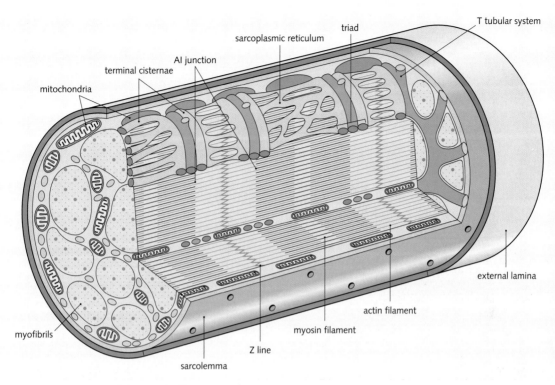

Fig. 2.10 Components of the muscle fiber.

Distribution of ions in the ICF and ECF of muscle cells		
Ion	**ICF (mmol/L)**	**ECF (mmol/L)**
Na⁺	12	145
K⁺	155	4
H⁺	13×10^{-5}	3.8×10^{-5}
Ca²⁺	8	1.5
Cl⁻	3.8	12.0
HCO³⁻	8	27
A⁻	155	0

Fig. 2.11 Distribution of ions in the intracellular fluid (ICF) and extracellular fluid (ECF) of muscle cells. A⁻, Organic impermeable anions (adapted from *Review of Medical Physiology*, 17th ed., by Ganong WF, Appleton & Lange, 1995).

The main ion responsible for the RMP is K^+. However, the RMP is not equal to the equilibrium potential of potassium (E_K), owing to:
- Small concentration of Na^+ leaking from ECF to ICF.
- Diffusion of Cl^-.
- Presence of protein-impermeable ions (A^-).
- The activities of the Na^+/K^+ pump.

Na⁺/K⁺ ATPase pump
Sites and functions
The Na^+/K^+ ATPase pump is found in the membranes of all body cells (see Fig. 2.12). Its functions are as follows:
- Maintenance of cell volume.
- Cotransport and countertransport of other solutes.

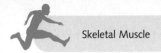
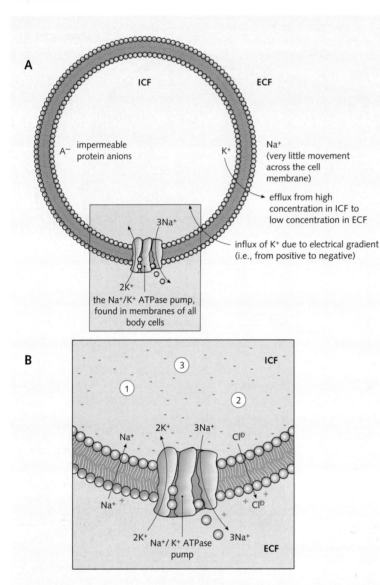

Fig. 2.12 Factors involved in the determination and maintenance of the resting membrane potential (RMP). K^+ is the key player. A. The Na^+ pump is found in membranes of all body cells. The mechanism of action is as follows: a removal of 3 Na^+ and an entry of 2 K^+ occur, expending 1 ATP molecule; phosphorylation of the protein subunits produces a conformational change and binding of Na^+; dephosphorylation results in binding of K^+ and reversion of the protein to its original shape. The cycle is repeated 100 times per second. Other contributors to RMP are shown in (B).
1. There is a passive leakage of a small amount of Na^+ from ECF to ICF along a concentration gradient.
2. Passive movement of Cl^- from ICF to ECF along an electrical gradient occurs.
3. A presence of impermeable protein anions (A^-) results. (Note that the bulk of the solution is electrochemically neutral. The excess ions close to the cell membrane are a small proportion. However, they are significant enough to cause movements across the cell membrane) (ICF, intracellular fluid; ECF, extracellular fluid).

- Contribution to RMP by maintaining the necessary electrostatic gradient (RMP is mainly due to passive K^+ efflux).
- Maintenance of the intracellular environment.

Mechanism of action

The removal of $3Na^+$ and entry of $2K^+$ expends an ATP molecule. Phosphorylation of the ATP protein subunits results in a conformational change and binding of Na^+, whereas dephosphorylation results in K^+ binding, which causes the protein to revert back to its original shape. This cycle is repeated 100 times per second (Fig. 2.13).

Electrochemical equilibrium

Electrochemical equilibrium (E) of K^+ is achieved when the forces acting in both directions are equal so that there is no net movement of K^+.

Equilibrium potential

Equilibrium potential is the voltage required to stop the diffusion of a permeable ion across the cell membrane. It can be calculated from the Nernst equation, given that the ion is permeable to the cell membrane and assuming that the Nernst potential is the potential inside the membrane and that the potential outside the

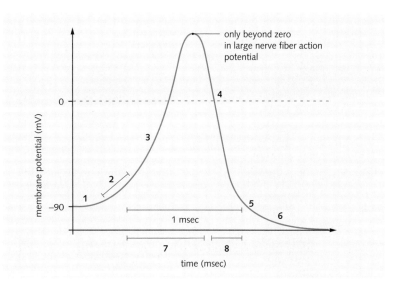

Fig. 2.13 Phases of the action potential (AP). (1) Resting membrane potential; (2) initial slow depolarization of cell in response to stimulus; (3) opening of voltage-gated Na^+ channels when threshold is reached; (4) repolarization (i.e., opening of voltage-gated K^+ channels); (5) return to resting membrane potential (−90 mV); (6) hyperpolarization due to "excessive" K^+ efflux; (7) absolute refractory period (AP may not be initiated); (8) relative refractory period (greater stimulus than normal to initiate the AP).

membrane is zero. The Nernst equation reads as follows:

$$E_{ion} = \frac{\pm\ 61\ \log\ [ion]_{ECF}}{\log\ [ion]_{ICF}}$$

In this equation, E is the equilibrium potential of the ion. The constant 61 takes into account the valency of the ion (Z), the absolute temperature (T), the gas constant (R), and the electrical constant (F). The [ion] represents the ion concentration in millimole per liter. Note that E_K is −95 mV, which is close to the value of a muscle cell's RMP, implying that the cell membrane is mainly permeable to K^+.

Effects of Na^+ and K^+ channels on the membrane potential
Depolarization
Depolarization results from the opening of Na^+ channels and an Na^+ influx. It results in a membrane potential that is less negative than the RMP.

Hyperpolarization
Hyperpolarization occurs upon closure of Na^+ channels and opening of K^+ channels, causing a K^+ efflux that restores, and may exceed, the normal RMP. This results in a membrane potential that is more negative than the RMP.

Action potential
An action potential (AP) is a transient depolarization of the cell membrane beyond a critical level or "threshold potential" (Fig. 2.14). When there is slow depolarization of a cell in response to a stimulus, an

AP is generated at the threshold potential via the triggering of voltage-gated ion channels. It is an important means of transmitting information through the nervous system and initiating contraction of muscle cells. The size and duration of the AP in different cell types vary.

Initiation of the AP
APs are usually initiated:
• At synapses—specialized junctions between cells.
• By the passage of current from one cell to another via gap junctions.

Both of these stimuli can activate a slow depolarization of the cell membrane, which reaches the critical threshold level and thus generates an AP. The all-or-none law states that once an AP has been initiated, the size is constant for a given type of cell and will not be affected by altering the stimuli strength.

Ionic basis of the AP
Both Na^+ and K^+ movements across the cell membrane are important (see Fig. 2.14). At rest, the voltage-activated Na^+ and K^+ channels are closed, although K^+ moves passively along a concentration gradient through the cell membrane.

Early phase of depolarization
During the early phase of depolarization, the fast gate (m-gate) of a voltage-gated Na^+ channel opens, and the slow gate (h-gate) starts to close. Since the slow gate takes longer to close, there is an influx of Na^+. This influx results in the activation of more Na^+

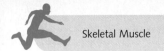

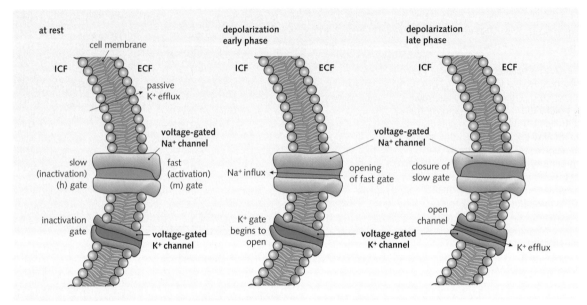

Fig. 2.14 Changes in voltage-activated channels during an action potential derived from studies using the voltage clamp and selective channel blockers (ICF, intracellular fluid;

channels via a feedback mechanism. The voltage-activated K^+ channel starts to open slowly.

Late phase of depolarization
During the late phase of depolarization, the slow gate of a voltage-gated Na^+ channel is closed, and there is no more influx of Na^+. The slow gate reopens when RMP is reached (i.e., when the fast gate is closed).

The K^+ channel is open and remains so until RMP is restored. Closure of the K^+ channel is slow, meaning that hyperpolarization may occur following an AP.

Propagation of the AP
An AP occurring at any one site on the cell membrane causes voltage changes in the adjacent parts of the membrane; these allow the AP to propagate in both directions. These changes can be explained by the local circuit theory (Fig. 2.15).

Saltatory conduction
Saltatory conduction occurs in myelinated nerve fibers (Fig. 2.16). The local circuit theory still applies, but the current can leave the axon only at the nodes of Ranvier. This results in a greater conduction velocity because the current density at the nodes is greater, so depolarization is more rapid.

The circuit of current can travel a number of internodal lengths and still be able to depolarize a

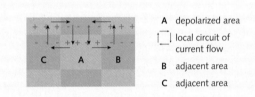

Fig. 2.15 Local circuit theory. The local circuit of current may cause sufficient depolarization in B and/or C to initiate an action potential. This can then be propagated in the same way.

node to threshold. This conserves energy for the axon, because only the nodes depolarize, allowing a minimal loss of ions and therefore requiring little metabolism for re-establishing the sodium and potassium concentration differences across the membrane after a series of nerve impulses.

Conduction velocity
In nerves, the conduction velocity (CV) ranges from 100 m/sec to less than 1 m/sec.

Factors affecting CV are as follows:
- Fiber diameter (i.e., myelin sheath, large nerve fibers): increasing the fiber diameter increases the conduction velocity.
- Temperature: increasing temperature increases the conduction velocity. Above 40°C, however,

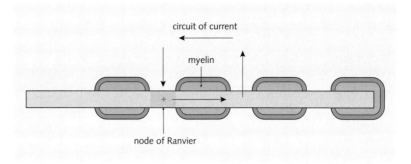

Fig. 2.16 Saltatory conduction in myelinated nerve fibers. The current is only able to leave at the nodes of Ranvier. The circuit of current can be thought of as "jumping" from node to node, allowing a greater speed of conduction.

Comparison of electrical and chemical synapses		
Property	**Electrical**	**Chemical**
Site	Nerves, heart, smooth muscle, liver, epithelium	Most of synapses in body, including skeletal muscle and brain
Structures seen at synapse	Gap junctions	Presynaptic vesicles and mitochondria, postsynaptic receptors
Mechanism of transmission	Ionic current	Chemical messenger
Cytoplasmic continuity between presynaptic and postsynaptic cell	Yes	No
Synaptic cleft	3.5 nm	20–40 nm
Nature of transmission	Rapid, usually excitatory effect on target cell	Synaptic delay 1–5 msec, excitatory or inhibitory effect on target cell
Plasticity	No	Yes
Amplification of signal	No	Yes

Fig. 2.17 Comparison of electrical and chemical synapses (adapted from *Human Physiology and Mechanisms of Disease*, 8th ed., by Guyton AC, W.B. Saunders, 1991).

the conduction velocity decreases until there is "heat block."
- Strength of local circuits: stronger local circuits result in a greater conduction velocity.

The synapse

The junction at which nerve cells communicate with each other is called a synapse. Synapses can be electrical or chemical. Electrical synapses direct transmission of current from a presynaptic cell to a target cell through ion channels. Chemical synapses release a chemical that binds to protein receptors on the target cell membrane, causing direct or indirect opening of ion channels (Fig. 2.17).

Transmission of a signal at a chemical synapse involves:
- An AP propagated at the presynaptic nerve terminal.
- Depolarization of the nerve terminal.
- Open voltage-activated Ca^{2+} channels, causing an influx of Ca^{2+}.
- Vesicles in the active zone fusing with the presynaptic membrane, releasing neurotransmitter by exocytosis.
- The neurotransmitter binding to protein receptors in the postsynaptic membrane.
- Changes in the postsynaptic membrane, leading to depolarization or hyperpolarization of the target cell.

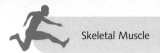

Electrical synapses correspond to gap junctions between certain cells (e.g., neurons, cardiac muscle cells, smooth muscle cells, epithelial cells). Transmission of a signal at an electrical synapse involves:

- Depolarization of the presynaptic membrane.
- Direct flow of current through gap junction ion channels to the target cell.
- Depolarization of the target cell.

Local anesthetics

Local anesthetics are drugs that are used to provide temporary relief of pain. They are weak bases: 90% are unionized and can cross the cell membrane but are not very effective at blocking the Na^+ channels, while 10% are ionized and block the Na^+ channels from inside the axon when the channels are open. The more common local anesthetics include lidocaine, bupivacaine, prilocaine, benzocaine, and cocaine.

Vasoconstrictors (e.g., epinephrine) are often administered with local anesthetics. The constricted blood vessels prevent too much local anesthetic from diffusing away from the relevant site, resulting in a longer duration of action and lower chance of systemic toxicity. However, the vasoconstrictors are never used in sites with small blood vessels (e.g., fingers, ears), owing to the risk of tissue ischemia resulting from vasospasm.

Mechanism of action

Local anesthetics block Na^+ channels to prevent depolarization and propagation of APs. The unionized form crosses the cell membrane, and 10% ionizes in the cytoplasm. This ionized form then blocks open Na^+ channels from within. Nerve fibers with a small diameter are more easily blocked; hence, local anesthetics can prevent the sensation of pain without affecting touch.

Use dependency

The more a nerve is stimulated, the greater the block achieved, because the Na^+ channels are blocked when open.

Adverse effects

Local anesthetics can affect the cardiovascular system by causing hypotension or cardiac arrest; they can also affect the central nervous system (CNS) by causing restlessness, sleepiness, convulsions, and respiratory depression. Anaphylaxis can also occur.

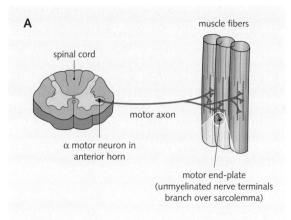

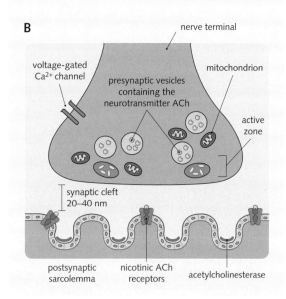

Fig. 2.18 Diagram demonstrating (A) the motor end plate and (B) the structure of the neuromuscular junction at a chemical synapse (ACh, acetylcholine).

Neuromuscular junction
Structure of the neuromuscular junction

At the neuromuscular junction (NMJ) each muscle fiber is innervated by one motor nerve (Fig. 2.18). The axon of each motor neuron divides into many branches as it enters the muscle, each branch forming an NMJ with a single muscle fiber. Each muscle fiber has only one NMJ.

The nerve terminal invaginates into the muscle fiber near its midpoint to form a depression in the muscle membrane, termed the synaptic trough (gutter). However, the nerve terminal does not cross the muscle membrane.

The synaptic cleft is the space between the nerve terminal and the muscle membrane. This cleft is occupied by connective tissue and ECF.

Presynaptic nerve terminal
Vesicles
At the presynaptic nerve terminal, acetylcholine (ACh) is synthesized in the cytoplasm and then stored in vesicles (about 10,000 molecules per vesicle) with an ATP molecule. At rest, 85% of ACh is stored in the vesicles, and 15% is present in the cytoplasm.

Mitochondria
Numerous mitochondria provide energy for the uptake of choline and synthesis of ACh.

Active zones
Active zones are specialized regions of the presynaptic membrane. They are sites of neurotransmitter release and are positioned so they lie opposite a junctional fold in the postsynaptic membrane.

Voltage-activated Ca^{2+} channels
Voltage-activated Ca^{2+} channels are believed to be adjacent to active zones. The channels open in response to an AP. The associated influx of Ca^{2+} causes the vesicles to move to the active zone.

Although the overall intracellular concentration of Ca^{2+} is relatively low, remember that there is a high concentration of Ca^{2+} in the sarcoplasmic reticulum.

Postsynaptic membrane
Motor end plate
The motor end plate is a specialized region of the muscle fiber membrane at which the terminal branches of the motor nerve communicate with the muscle fiber.

Junctional folds
Junctional folds are folds in the motor end plate on which nicotinic ACh receptors (nicAChR) are located. These folds increase the surface area on which the transmitter can act.

Basal lamina
The basal lamina is connective tissue lying between the nerve terminal and muscle fiber membrane. Large quantities of the enzyme acetylcholinesterase are found here, particularly at the bases of the junctional folds.

Nicotinic ACh receptor
The nicAChR consists of five protein subunits (2α, 1β, 1γ, and 1δ). The binding of two ACh molecules (one to each of the two α subunits) induces a conformational change, and the channel opens. The channel is permeable to both K^+ and Na^+. However, concentration gradients favor Na^+ influx.

When a nerve AP arrives at the NMJ, a sequence of events takes place and lasts only 10–15 msec. This sequence is numbered to correspond to Fig. 2.19, as follows:
1. The AP arrives at the nerve terminal.
2. The voltage-activated Ca^{2+} channels open, allowing Ca^{2+} influx.
3. Ca^{2+} influx attracts presynaptic vesicles to the active zones.
4. Vesicles fuse to the presynaptic membrane and release ACh in "packets" by the process of exocytosis.
5. ACh diffuses across the synaptic cleft to bind to nicAChR on the junctional folds. Activation of channels and an influx of Na^+ occur.
6. Na^+ influx depolarizes the muscle. This is called an end-plate potential (epp). The epp depolarizes adjacent regions of the muscle membrane. Upon reaching the threshold, an AP occurs in the muscle fiber.
7. Rapid removal of ACh from the synaptic trough terminates the activation of the receptors. This removal occurs in two ways: (1) the action of acetylcholinesterase hydrolyzes ACh to choline and acetic acid; (2) a small amount of ACh that has diffused out of the trough is broken down by pseudocholinesterase in the plasma.
8. Uptake of choline into nerve terminals is the rate-limiting step of ACh synthesis. This is an active process requiring the hydrolysis of ATP and involves two carrier systems: the high affinity–low capacity mechanism, which is responsible for 90% of the uptake, and the low affinity–high capacity mechanism.
9. Recycled choline reacts with acetyl CoA (formed in the mitochondria and transported into the cytoplasm). The enzyme choline acetyltransferase

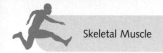

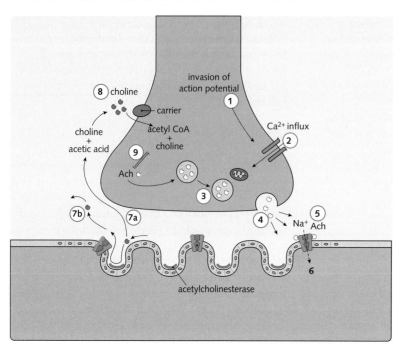

Fig. 2.19 Events at the neuromuscular junction upon arrival of a nerve action potential. Refer to the text for an explanation of the sequence (which occurs in 10–15 msec) (ACh, acetylcholine).

Comparison of the action potential of skeletal muscle with nerve		
Property	**Skeletal muscle AP**	**Nerve AP**
RMP	–80 to –90 mV	–40 mV (small nerves) to –90 mV (large nerves)
Duration	1–5 msec	<1 msec
Spread of AP to interior	T tubule system	Depolarization of membrance is sufficient
Conduction velocity	3 5 m/sec	<1–100 msec, depends on a number of factors

Fig. 2.20 Comparison of the action potential (AP) in skeletal muscle with the AP in nerves.

catalyzes the reaction. The vesicle membrane is also recycled by endocytosis from the nerve terminal membrane. ACh is again stored in "packets" in the nerve terminal.

AP in skeletal muscle
The ionic basis of the AP in skeletal muscle is the same as the AP in nerves. However, there are certain differences between the two (Fig. 2.20).

Drugs acting at the NMJ
Drugs acting presynaptically
Hemicholinium acts presynaptically at the NMJ by blocking the uptake of choline. There is a slow

depletion of ACh in the nerve terminal. Aminoglycosides and botulinum toxin inhibit ACh release.

Drugs enhancing transmission
Anticholinesterases enhance transmission at the NMJ by increasing the time that ACh is present in the synaptic cleft.

Mechanism of action: Anticholinesterases inhibit acetylcholinesterase. There are three main types of anticholinesterases: short-acting (up to 15 minutes) drugs (e.g, edrophonium), which bind reversibly to the active site of the enzyme; intermediate-acting drugs (e.g., pyridostigmine and neostigmine), which bind covalently to the enzyme; and long-acting drugs (e.g., organophosphorus compounds), which form strong covalent bonds with the active site. Long-acting drugs are often referred to as irreversible because the enzyme is inactivated for a long period of time; they have no clinical use but are used in chemical weapons.

Indications: Edrophonium assists in the diagnosis of myasthenia gravis. An intravenous injection leads to short-term improvement in muscle strength. Treatment involves the use of intermediate-acting anticholinesterases. Anticholinesterases reverse competitive neuromuscular block after surgery.

Adverse effects: Side effects of anticholinesterases include paradoxical depolarizing neuromuscular block; convulsions, coma, and respiratory arrest if a lipid-soluble anticholinesterase (e.g., physostigmine) is used; and symptoms associated with the parasympathetic nervous system, because ACh is the neurotransmitter acting on muscarinic receptors.

Drugs acting postsynaptically
Neuromuscular-blocking drugs are either competitive or depolarizing.

Competitive drugs
Tubocurarine and gallamine are examples of competitive neuromuscular-blocking drugs.

Mechanism of action: Neuromuscular-blocking drugs compete with ACh for binding sites on the ACh receptor in the postsynaptic membrane. There is no opening of the ion channel when they bind; therefore, AP generation in muscle is less likely. Their action is reversed by anticholinesterases and enhanced by general anesthetics.

Indications: Neuromuscular-blocking drugs are used in surgery to relax skeletal muscles and are used for electroconvulsive therapy.

Adverse effects: Side effects of neuromuscular-blocking drugs include a decrease in blood pressure (owing to blockage of autonomic nicotinic receptors) and anaphylaxis.

Depolarizing drugs
Suxamethonium is an example of a depolarizing drug.

Mechanism of action: Depolarizing drugs are nicotinic agonists with blockage that occurs because of prolonged membrane depolarization and desensitization of nicotinic receptors. Their action is potentiated by anticholinesterases.

Indications: Depolarizing drugs are used in surgery to relax skeletal muscles and are used for electroconvulsive therapy. Although competitive blockers are more widely used, depolarizing drugs tend to be used for brief procedures.

Adverse effects: Because initial stimulation occurs before blockage, asynchronous muscle fiber twitches may result in muscle pains following the use of depolarizing drugs. Other side effects include bradycardia due to action on muscarinic receptors.

Excitation–contraction coupling
Excitation–contraction coupling refers to the events that occur from initiation of an AP in the sarcolemma to contraction of muscle and subsequent relaxation.

Initiation of an AP in muscle fiber
The epp resulting from a single neuronal AP is usually greater in amplitude than that required to initiate an AP in muscle fiber. For this reason, the NMJ is said to have a very high "safety factor."

Propagation of an AP into muscle fiber via T tubules
An AP is propagated into muscle fiber via T tubules in a sequence of events (the following numbers refer to Fig. 2.21).
1. Bidirectional propagation of the AP occurs along the sarcolemma. This causes excitation of muscle fiber along its whole length so that all sarcomeres contract simultaneously.
2. The AP is then propagated into the muscle fiber via the T tubule. There are two T tubules per sarcomere. These encircle the myofibril at the AI junction. T tubules communicate with the extracellular space.
3. The sarcoplasmic reticulum on both sides of the T tubule communicates with the T tubule via junctional feet. Depolarization of the T tubule results in a signal from the T tubule to the sarcoplasmic reticulum terminal cisternae.
4. Ca^{2+} channels then open in the sarcoplasmic reticulum, and Ca^{2+} moves along a concentration gradient into the sarcoplasm around the myofibrils.

Muscle contraction
Two types of molecule—thick and thin filaments—are involved in muscle contraction (Fig. 2.22).

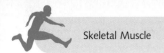
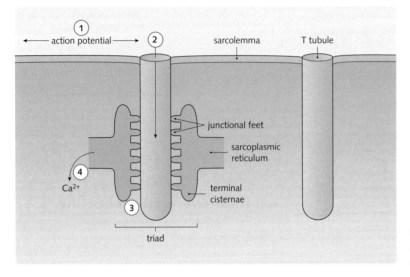

Fig. 2.21 Sarcoplasmic release of intracellular Ca^{2+}. The numbers refer to the text.

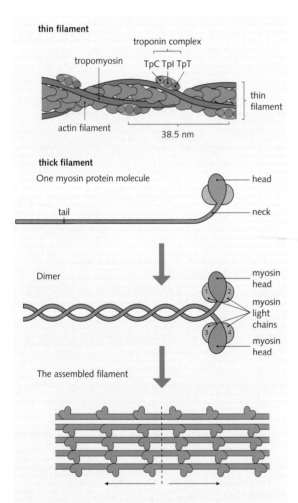

Fig. 2.22 Different arrangement of contractile proteins in thin filament and thick (myosin) filament.

Thick filament

Myosin: This is the main component of thick filament. It is a much larger protein than actin and consists of a tail, neck, and head (cross-bridge) region.

The head region possesses ATPase activity and can attach to specific binding sites on the actin molecule; the neck region is flexible, which is necessary for attachment and detachment to the actin filament, and the tail region provides strength.

Thin filament

Actin: This is the main component of thin filament. It is capable of binding five other proteins.

Tropomyosin: This is a structural protein that can bind to actin filaments. Each tropomyosin binds to seven actin filaments. Tropomyosin "covers" the myosin-binding sites on the actin filament, thereby preventing a myosin–actin interaction.

Troponin: This protein consists of a complex of three subunits: T, which binds one tropomyosin; C, which has a high affinity for Ca^{2+}; and I, which has a high affinity for actin (hence the attachment of tropomyosin to actin). The binding of Ca^{2+} causes a change in shape and movement of the associated tropomyosin, which uncovers the myosin attachment site on actin.

α-Actinin: This protein is found in the Z band.

Mechanism of contraction
Huxley's cross-bridge cycle

Huxley's cross-bridge cycle demonstrates the shortening of the sarcomere caused by the sliding

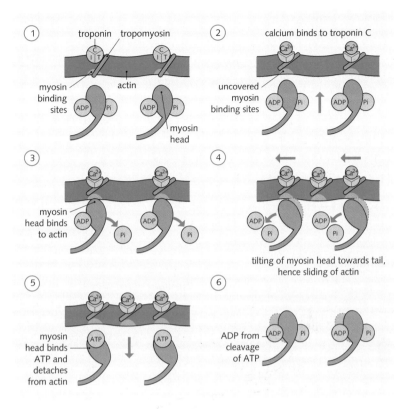

Fig. 2.23 Interaction of myosin heads with thin filaments during contraction. The numbers refer to the text.

of the actin filaments. The numbers correspond to Fig. 2.23 as follows:

1. In the resting state, the myosin attachment sites on the actin molecule are covered by tropomyosin.
2. An increase in intracellular Ca^{2+} results in the binding of Ca^{2+} to troponin C. The binding of Ca^{2+} causes a conformational change in the troponin complex, resulting in movement of the tropomyosin and uncovering of the myosin binding sites.
3. The myosin head attaches to an actin molecule and releases the phosphate group.
4. This attachment causes the myosin head to tilt toward its tail, thereby pulling the actin filament in that direction. Tilting of the head causes release of adenosine diphosphate (ADP).
5. A molecule of ATP binds to the myosin head. This causes detachment of the head from the actin.
6. The ATPase action of the myosin head cleaves ATP, resulting in a myosin head with attached ADP and phosphate. The energy derived from this process causes straightening

(or "untilting") of the head, preparing it for reattachment.

The whole process is then repeated. In this way, the myosin head "walks" along the actin filament. This is the basis of the "walk along" theory.

Relaxation of muscle

Relaxation of muscle is dependent on Ca^{2+}. Upon repolarization of the muscle fiber, Ca^{2+} is actively pumped back into the sarcoplasmic reticulum. The concentration of Ca^{2+} drops, and it is no longer bound to troponin. The myosin-binding sites become "covered" by tropomyosin again, preventing further "walking."

Bioenergetics of muscle contraction

Muscle contraction results in energy expenditure during:

- Interaction of actin and myosin filaments during contraction.
- Pumping of Ca^{2+} from the sarcoplasm back into the sarcoplasmic reticulum after contraction.
- Restoration of the intracellular ionic environment after muscle contraction because of the actions of the Na^+/K^+ pump.

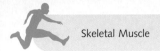

Sources of energy
Short-term sources
Sarcoplasm: ATP molecules are present in sarcoplasm. These would be expended within the first 2 seconds of contraction if they were not replaced.

Creatine phosphokinase: As a substrate, creatine phosphokinase contains high-energy phosphate bonds, which can be used to phosphorylate ADP to ATP by the enzyme creatine kinase. It is located in the Z line.

Myokinase: The enzyme myokinase catalyzes the transfer of a phosphate group from one ADP molecule to another to form ATP and the by-product adenosine monophosphate (AMP).

Intermediate-term sources
Anaerobic glycolysis: This type of glycolysis causes the breakdown of glucose to lactate and pyruvate with the release of energy, which is used to convert ADP to ATP. ATP is generated at double the rate of oxidative phosphorylation. See *Crash Course: Metabolism and Nutrition* for more detail.

Anaerobic glycolysis is predominant in type II muscle fibers that have few mitochondria but many glycogen granules. This is only an intermediate-term source of energy, because lactate and pyruvate accumulate in the cell.

Long-term sources
Oxidative phosphorylation: This type of phosphorylation is an aerobic process in which ATP is liberated from fats, carbohydrates, and protein. See *Crash Course: Metabolism and Nutrition* for more information.

Energy can be provided for longer periods (a few hours) than with glycolysis. Type I muscle fibers are suited to oxidative phosphorylation because they have numerous mitochondria and lipid droplets.

Myofiber cytoskeleton
The myofiber cytoskeleton is essential to the mechanical stability and function of muscle. The proteins present in the myofiber cytoskeleton are dystrophin and bridging glycoproteins.

Actin filaments are linked to dystrophin, which in turn is linked to a number of glycoproteins that extend to the surface of the sarcolemma. These glycoproteins link to laminin in the basement membrane (Fig. 2.24).

The myofiber cytoskeleton forms a link between the inside of the cell and the extracellular matrix. (The extracellular matrix supports the muscle fiber,

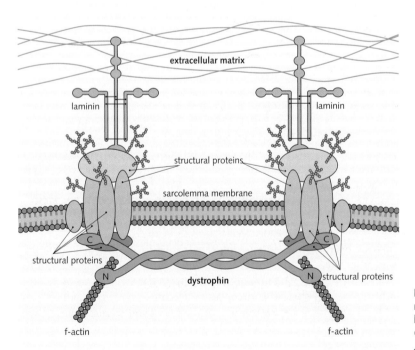

Fig. 2.24 Components of the myofiber cytoskeleton and their linkage with the extracellular matrix (adapted from *Muscle and Nerve* by J. Wiley and Sons, 1994).

decreasing the likelihood of tearing upon contraction.) Duchenne muscular dystrophy is an example of a condition resulting from abnormalities in the myofiber cytoskeleton.

Functions of skeletal muscle

Motor unit

The motor unit refers to the motor neuron (lower motor neuron) and all the muscle fibers innervated by it.

Each motor neuron may innervate many muscle fibers, but a single muscle fiber receives input from only one motor neuron.

The number of muscle fibers innervated by a motor neuron is known as the "innervation ratio." A smaller number of muscle fibers per motor neuron is present in muscles involved in fine, precise movements (e.g., ocular muscles), while a larger number is seen in muscles involved in gross movements (e.g., maintaining posture).

The muscle fibers innervated by a single motor neuron are spread out in the muscle.

The muscle fibers in a motor unit are of the same type and contract simultaneously.

There are three different types of motor units (Fig. 2.25).

Orderly recruitment

Small motor neurons innervate slow muscle fibers (type I), whereas larger motor neurons innervate fast muscle fibers (types IIa and IIb). This is referred to as the size principle.

Smaller motor neurons require a smaller excitatory input for activation. During reflex or voluntary movement for a given excitatory input, the slow units are activated first. This results in an orderly recruitment of muscle fibers, with activation of slow units first, followed by activation of fast fatigue-resistant units and, finally, of fast fatigable units. This is important *in vivo* because it allows movement to be graded by altering the level of excitatory input rather than having to select different fiber types.

Effects of denervation and reinnervation on motor units

Denervation of a motor unit (lower motor neuron lesion) results in atrophy of the muscle fibers in that unit. There may also be fibrillations on the electromyogram, shown as fine, irregular contractions of individual fibers, and an increase in sensitivity to circulating ACh.

Clinically, the signs of a lower motor neuron lesion are apparent in patients. These include muscle wasting, a decrease in muscle tone, decrease

Properties of different motor unit types			
Property	**Motor unit type**		
	Slow, resistant to fatigue	Fast, nonfatigable	Fast, fatigable
Fiber diameter	Small (type I)	Intermediate (type IIa)	Large (type IIb)
Force of contraction	Low	Intermediate	High
Myosin–ATPase activity (indicates rate of ATP hydrolysis and therefore speed of twitch)	Low	Low	High
Source of energy	Oxidative phosphorylation	Oxidative phosphorylation and some anaerobic glycolysis	Anaerobic glycolysis
Glycogen content	Low	Intermediate	High
Mitochondria	Many	Many	Few
Capillaries	Many	Many	Few
Function	Fine movement and maintenance of posture	Sustained activity	Brief, strong contractions (e.g., jumping)

Fig. 2.25 Properties of different motor unit types.

in or loss of power of contraction, and diminished tendon reflexes.

Some of the muscle fibers are replaced by fibrous and fatty tissue. However, this fibrous tissue shortens, and contractures may form.

Other muscle fibers may be reinnervated by collaterals from the remaining adjacent motor neurons. This results in:

- Possible alteration of the fiber type because the motor neuron determines the fiber type. There may be areas of muscle containing fibers of only one type, which is termed fiber clumping and produces characteristic waveforms on a diagnostic electromyogram (EMG).
- Larger motor units.

Muscle mechanics
Isometric contraction
Isometric contraction occurs in muscle with a constant length. Isometric tests can be used to compare force against duration of contraction of different muscles (Figs. 2.26 and 2.27).

Isotonic contraction
Isotonic contraction occurs in muscle with a constant tension. The length of the muscle changes while maintaining constant tension. Isotonic tests can be used to compare the speed of shortening of different muscle types (see Fig. 2.27).

Sarcoplasmic Ca^{2+} concentration and muscle twitch
Every AP in skeletal muscle results in a similar amount of Ca^{2+} release. Hence, under isometric conditions, the force of the twitch resulting from a single AP will remain the same.

Unlike myocardium, the strength of contraction in skeletal muscle is not dependent on sarcoplasmic Ca^{2+} concentration, because each AP results in sufficient Ca^{2+} release to produce the maximal response.

Maximal response in skeletal muscle, however, is not seen with a single AP because:
- Series elasticity occurs, whereby structural components (e.g., tendons, cross-bridges) of the muscle are elastic and lengthen when force is generated; therefore, initial shortening of muscle is slow.
- Sarcoplasmic Ca^{2+} is rapidly pumped back into the sarcoplasmic reticulum following an AP, thereby ending the response.

Force of contraction in skeletal muscle may be increased by maintaining the sarcoplasmic Ca^{2+} concentration by repetitive stimulation. This would result in greater shortening—the initial twitch would be involved in stretching of the elastic elements with no "wasting" of force upon subsequent twitches because the elastic elements are already stretched (Fig. 2.28).

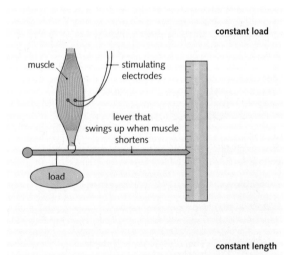

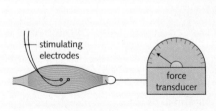

Fig. 2.27 Measurement of isotonic and isometric contractions (modified from *Human Physiology and Mechanisms of Disease*, 8th ed., by Guyton AC, W.B. Saunders, 1992).

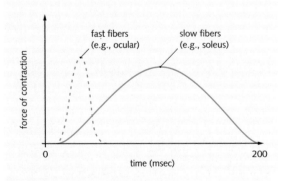

Fig. 2.26 Duration of contraction in different muscles demonstrated by isometric tests.

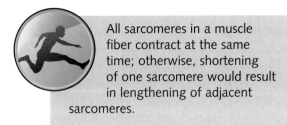

All sarcomeres in a muscle fiber contract at the same time; otherwise, shortening of one sarcomere would result in lengthening of adjacent sarcomeres.

Maintained muscle contractions

Twitch is a single contraction resulting from a single AP. It is a submaximal response. Unfused tetanus occurs when muscle is repetitively stimulated, which does not allow sufficient time for complete relaxation between each twitch. As a result, the successive mechanical responses fuse, with an additive effect on force of contraction. This is called summation of twitches (Fig. 2.29).

Fused tetanus results from summation of twitches. However, there is no relaxation of muscle between each stimulus, resulting in fusion of consecutive twitches and a smooth sustained contraction.

Summation of twitches is an important means of varying the force of contraction. Therefore, increasing the frequency of stimulation is an important means of modulating force of contraction (see Fig. 2.29).

Tetany is spasm and twitching of skeletal muscle due to low levels of extracellular Ca^{2+}. A decrease in extracellular Ca^{2+} lowers the threshold for activation of muscle and nerve cells. This is not the same as a tetanus, which is a normal feature of skeletal muscle.

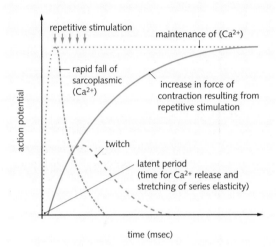

Fig. 2.28 Relationship of sarcoplasmic (Ca^{2+}) to force of contraction in skeletal muscle. Repeat stimulation results in maintenance of intracellular Ca^{2+}. Series elasticity refers to the inherent elasticity of muscle tissue, including its noncontractile C/T matrix. The latent period can be thought of as "taking up the slack" before contraction of the tissue begins. In repetitive stimulation, the elastic elements remain stretched, improving muscle efficiency (adapted from *Physiology*, 3rd ed., by Berne RM and Levy MN, Mosby Year Book, 1993).

Length–tension relationship

The force or tension a muscle fiber generates depends on the length of the sarcomere (Fig. 2.30). There is an optimum range of lengths at which the force generated is at its maximum. This can be explained by the sliding filament theory—if a sarcomere is stretched, the overlap between actin and myosin is reduced, and there are fewer

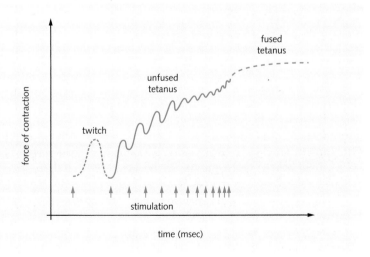

Fig. 2.29 Summation of twitches. As the time between each twitch decreases, the force of the contraction increases, showing the modulating effect of stimulation frequency.

33

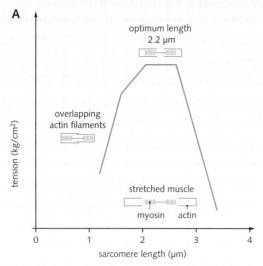

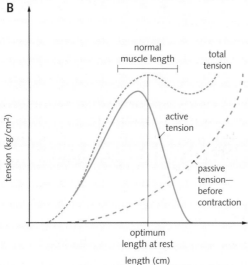

Fig. 2.30 A. Effect of sarcomere length on the active tension developed by an individual muscle fiber upon contraction. B. Effect of muscle length on tension. Increasing the passive tension initially increases the total tension. Further increases in passive tension lead to a decrease in active tension.

actin–myosin interactions and lower force. Alternatively, if the sarcomere is shortened, the thin filaments overlap and the number of actin–myosin interactions are again reduced.

In a whole muscle, the total tension developed is the sum of active tension and passive tension:

- Total tension results from isometric contraction of muscle in response to a maximal stimulus.
- Passive tension results from stretching of the muscle in the absence of contraction and is caused by the elastic forces of connective tissue,

blood vessels, and other such physiologic elements.

- Active tension is the increase in tension resulting from muscular contraction. This is determined by subtracting passive tension from total tension. Most muscles in the body are at the optimum length for maximum tension.

Modulation of skeletal muscle contraction force

Force of muscle contraction is modulated by orderly recruitment and increasing frequency of stimulation. Other important factors include the length of the muscle and the influence of the antagonistic muscle groups.

Force–velocity relationship

The force–velocity relationship is found by stimulating a muscle under isotonic conditions and measuring the speed of shortening with different loads. The speed of shortening is decreased with increasing loads (Fig. 2.31, A).

Speed of shortening varies with different fiber types. This occurs because of the existence of myosin isoforms. In fast fibers, myosin ATPase activity is rapid; therefore, cross-bridge cycling and shortening of muscle fibers are more rapid (Fig. 2.31, B). The speed of shortening is inversely related to the load.

Power curves

The power of muscle contraction is influenced by the speed of shortening (velocity) and the load (Fig. 2.32):

$$Power = velocity \times load$$

Although increasing the load would seem to favor the equation, this is not the case; increasing the load would decrease the speed of shortening. Hence, maximal power is actually achieved by a balance between the load and the speed of shortening.

Muscle plasticity

Muscle plasticity refers to changes in the characteristics of a muscle to match function. Factors that may be altered include muscle fiber diameter, length, strength, and vascular supply.

The fiber types may also be altered but to a lesser extent because they are determined by the motor neuron by which they are innervated.

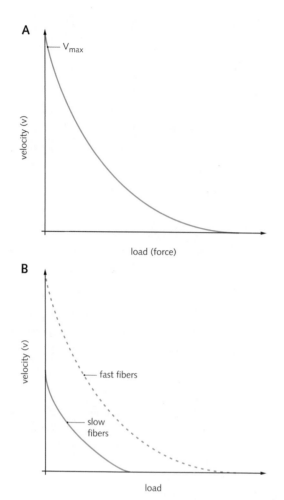

Fig. 2.31 Graphs showing speeds of contraction. A. Speed of contraction that decreases with increasing load, with maximum velocity occurring with zero load. B. Maximum speed of contraction in fast fibers greater than the speed in slow fibers.

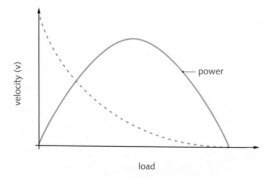

Fig. 2.32 Maximal power resulting from a balance between speed of shortening and load.

Fast fibers are interconvertible (i.e., fast glycolytic fibers may be converted to fast oxidative and vice versa). Slow and fast fibers are not interconvertible.

Effect of exercise on muscle

An increase in muscle mass can result from hypertrophy or hyperplasia. Hypertrophy of muscle is an increase in the size of individual muscle fibers, resulting in an increase in the force of contraction. This is caused by regular contraction of the muscle at maximal force.

Hyperplasia of muscle occurs to a lesser extent than does hypertrophy. Hyperplasia involves an increase in the number of muscle cells. This is not due to mitosis but rather to a splitting lengthwise of large fibers.

A lack of exercise causes muscle atrophy. This is a decrease in muscle fiber size resulting from lack of stimulation.

Relationship of muscle characteristics to function

Sprinters have a greater number of fast fibers because they require rapid contractions of large force, while marathon runners have a greater number of slow muscle fibers because they require sustained low-force contractions. The number of slow muscle fibers is largely genetically determined. By training, the effect of these muscle fibers may be enhanced by increasing their size and vascular supply.

Clinical relevance of muscle plasticity

Cardiomyoplasty involves the mobilizing of a skeletal muscle near to the heart, usually the latissimus dorsi. The skeletal muscle can then be wrapped around the heart to replace diseased or congenitally missing myocardium.

Individual skeletal muscle fibers may be regarded as a syncytium because each fiber is made up of a number of myoblasts that have fused. However, skeletal muscle fibers contract independently of each other; therefore, skeletal muscle is not referred to as a syncytium.

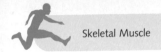
Disorders of skeletal muscle

Disorders of the neuromuscular junction

Disorders of the NMJ can be classified into two types: presynaptic or postsynaptic. Both types are associated with muscle weakness.

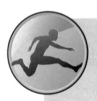 Disorders of the NMJ are not diseases of the muscle but rather disorders of function. Hence, atrophy tends to be a late feature.

Presynaptic abnormalities
Botulism
Etiology: Botulinum is an endotoxin produced by an organism called *Clostridium botulinum.*

Pathogenesis: Poisoning by botulinum is called botulism. Botulism is caused by the ingestion of canned meat contaminated with the endotoxin of *C. botulinum.* The endotoxin acts by blocking the uptake of choline at the NMJ.

Clinical features: Botulism causes symmetrical descending paralysis, particularly of the face and respiratory muscles. Signs include diplopia, loss of pupillary reflex, and laryngeal palsy.

Diagnosis: The diagnosis of botulism is clinical and is confirmed by detection of the endotoxin in food or in feces.

Management: Management of botulism involves supportive care and administration of antitoxin. Antibiotics may also be required.

Prognosis: There is an associated mortality rate of around 50% with botulism.

Lambert–Eaton myasthenic syndrome
The Lambert–Eaton myasthenic syndrome is a nonmetastatic complication of malignancy that involves antibodies to voltage-gated Ca^{2+} channels in the presynaptic membrane. The syndrome is most often associated with small-cell lung carcinomas. The malignant cells express Ca^{2+} channels and may trigger the formation of the antibodies.

When nerves are stimulated at the NMJ, there is a decrease in Ca^{2+} influx. This leads to a decrease in the release of ACh. Patients with Lambert–Eaton

myasthenic syndrome present with abnormal fatigability.

Postsynaptic abnormalities
Myasthenia gravis
Epidemiology: Symptoms of myasthenia gravis arise most commonly in the patient's third decade of life; the disease predominates in women and commonly presents between 20 and 40 years of age.

Etiology: The cause of myasthenia gravis is unknown. It may be due to recurrent viral illness resulting in the formation of antibodies.

Pathology: Myasthenia gravis is an autoimmune disease (Fig. 2.33). In 90% of patients, there are IgG antibodies to the ACh receptor in the postsynaptic membrane.

A decrease in functional ACh receptors results from:
• Stearic prevention of ACh binding to receptors because of the presence of antibody. The antibody does not itself bind to the ACh site but prevents ACh from binding.
• Increased breakdown of receptors.

Clinical features of myasthenia gravis
The main symptoms of myasthenia gravis are muscle weakness and fatigability. The ocular, bulbar, and cranial muscles are most commonly affected. Signs include ptosis and diplopia. The patient has generalized muscular weakness and may be in respiratory distress. Muscle bulk is maintained until late in the disease.

Myasthenia gravis is remitting and relapsing and symptoms worsen with exercise. Other autoimmune diseases (e.g., rheumatoid arthritis and systemic lupus erythematosus [SLE]) are often associated with myasthenia gravis. About 10% of patients have an associated thymoma, and almost half of patients show thymic hyperplasia. The heart is not affected.

Neonatal myasthenia may be seen in newborn babies of mothers with the disease. The babies present with poor limb movements and poor ability to feed. These symptoms last a few weeks until the maternal antibodies decrease.

Diagnosis of myasthenia gravis
About 90% of patients with myasthenia gravis have circulating anti-ACh receptor antibodies. Diagnosis is based on the Tensilon test (Fig. 2.34).

This test involves giving an injection of a short-acting anticholinesterase drug called edrophonium to

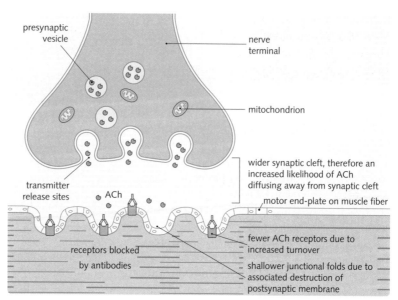

Fig. 2.33 Features of the neuromuscular junction in myasthenia gravis.

presynaptic vesicle

nerve terminal

mitochondrion

wider synaptic cleft, therefore an increased likelihood of ACh diffusing away from synaptic cleft

motor end-plate on muscle fiber

transmitter release sites

ACh

receptors blocked by antibodies

fewer ACh receptors due to increased turnover

shallower junctional folds due to associated destruction of postsynaptic membrane

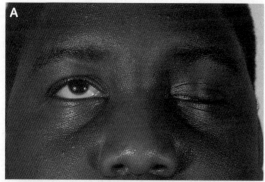

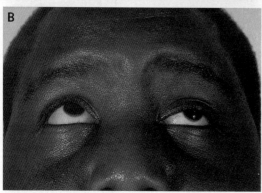

Fig. 2.34 The Tensilon test. A. Muscle weakness caused by repeated facial movements. B. Rapid improvement after administration of edrophonium, a short-acting anticholinesterase (courtesy of Dr. GD Perkin).

the suspected myasthenic patient. Because anticholinesterase drugs inhibit the enzyme acetylcholinesterase (which hydrolyzes ACh, thereby terminating the activation of ACh receptors on the muscle fiber), ACh is present in the synaptic cleft for a longer period of time, and there is a greater probability that it will bind to the ACh receptor. Therefore, muscle contraction can take place sufficiently for the patient to regain normal muscle strength temporarily. An EMG shows a decrease in response to stimulation.

Management and prognosis for a patient with myasthenia gravis

Management of a patient with myasthenia gravis involves the administration of long-lasting anticholinesterases—the dose varies according to the patient's response. Long-lasting anticholinesterases prolong the presence of ACh in the synaptic cleft, thereby increasing the likelihood of ACh binding to a receptor.

In patients with an associated thymoma, a thymectomy is needed. Administration of immunosuppressives, such as prednisolone or azathioprine, is also useful. As for the prognosis for these patients, the course of myasthenia gravis is variable. Death may result from aspiration pneumonia.

It is important to understand myasthenia gravis because it is a debilitating disease that is relatively common and may be challenging to manage effectively.

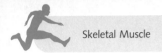
Inherited myopathies
Muscular dystrophies

The muscular dystrophies are a group of disorders involving a progressive degeneration of skeletal muscle.

X-linked dystrophies

Duchenne muscular dystrophy   *Epidemiology:* Duchenne muscular dystrophy occurs in 1 in 4000 live male births. One-third of the cases have no family history. Spontaneous mutations are likely because the gene involved is large.

Etiology: Duchenne muscular dystrophy is an X-linked recessive disorder.

Pathology: In Duchenne muscular dystrophy, a mutation occurs on the short arm of the X chromosome, the site (Xp21) coding for the dystrophin protein. The lack of the dystrophin protein results in impaired anchorage of muscle fibers to the extracellular matrix. This makes the muscle fibers more susceptible to tearing upon repeated contraction. Damaged fibers allow an influx of calcium ions, leading to irreversible cell death.

Clinical features: Children with Duchenne muscular dystrophy usually present at 2 years of age. Symptoms include weakness of the pelvic and shoulder girdle muscles; signs include selective atrophy, waddling gait, pseudohypertrophy of the calves, and Gowers' sign (Fig. 2.35).

Diagnosis: The average age for the diagnosis of Duchenne muscular dystrophy is 5 years. Diagnosis is based on a raised serum creatinine phosphokinase concentration. Muscle biopsy also reveals necrotic muscle fibers surrounded by fibrous tissue and fat (Fig. 2.36). The muscle fibers are of variable diameters, owing to the body's attempt at regeneration.

Complications: Complications of Duchenne muscular dystrophy include marked scoliosis, impaired learning (30%), contractures, and cardiomyopathy.

Management: There is no treatment that will halt Duchenne muscular dystrophy; management is supportive and is aimed at maintaining the use of the muscles and decreasing respiratory symptoms. Identification of female carriers is possible, and genetic counseling may be offered.

Prognosis: Most people with Duchenne muscular dystrophy are wheelchair-bound by their teens. Death occurs in the late teens or second decade of life and is due to cardiac failure or failure of the respiratory muscles.

Becker muscular dystrophy   Becker muscular dystrophy is a less common X-linked variant of

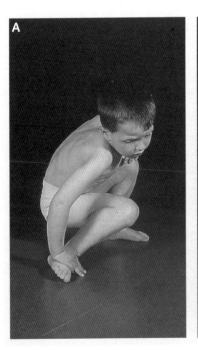
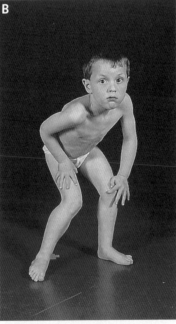

Fig. 2.35 Gowers' sign showing the difficulty encountered in standing from the prone position in patients with Duchenne muscular dystrophy. A. A child who needs to turn prone to rise and then uses his hands to climb upon his knees. B. Patient at knee level with hands being released and arms and trunk swung sideways and upward to reach an upright position. Note the hypertrophied calves (due to deposition of fat and fibrous tissue) (courtesy of Dr. T Lissauer and Dr. G Clayden).

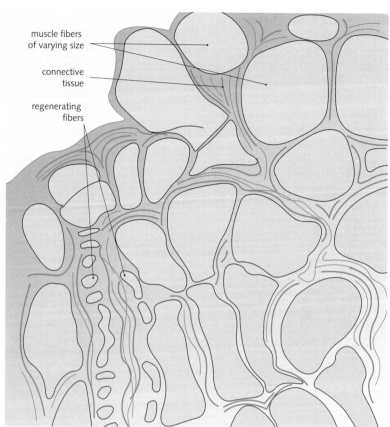

Fig. 2.36 Histologic changes in Duchenne muscular dystrophy showing variation in fiber diameter, increased fibrous and fatty connective tissue, and fiber generation.

muscle fibers of varying size

connective tissue

regenerating fibers

Duchenne muscular dystrophy. It shows similar clinical features to Duchenne muscular dystrophy, although the progression of the disease is slower. The average age of onset is 11 years with death occurring in the fourth decade of life.

 Of the inherited myopathies, Duchenne muscular dystrophy is a common topic in exams.

Autosomal dystrophies

Limb girdle dystrophy   Limb girdle dystrophy, one of the autosomal recessive dystrophies, presents in childhood or adulthood with pelvic and shoulder girdle weakness (Fig. 2.37).

Pseudohypertrophy of the calves is less common than in Duchenne muscular dystrophy. Muscle biopsy shows findings similar to those of Duchenne muscular dystrophy. Prognosis involves a variable degree of disability.

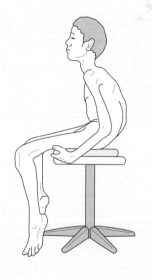

Fig. 2.37 Severe limb girdle dystrophy demonstrating proximal muscle wasting and kyphosis.

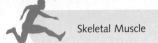

Facioscapulohumeral dystrophy   Facioscapulohumeral dystrophy is an autosomal dominant
disorder. The condition presents in childhood or
adulthood with face and shoulder girdle weakness.
Winging of the scapulae is characteristic.
Pseudohypertrophy is rare. Muscle biopsy shows
findings similar to those of Duchenne muscular
dystrophy. Individuals show a mild degree of
disability.

Myotonic disorders

Myotonic disorders are a group of conditions
in which there is a delay in muscle relaxation
after voluntary contraction. Administration of
general anesthetics is more likely to cause
complications in patients with muscle disorders
of this sort.

Myotonic dystrophy   *Epidemiology:* Myotonic
dystrophy occurs in 1 in 8000 people.

Etiology: Myotonic dystrophy is an autosomal
dominant disorder.

Pathology: The condition is caused by a mutation
on chromosome 19, the site coding for a cAMP-
dependent kinase. In affected families, the disease is
more severe in later generations. This is known as
anticipation.

Clinical features: Myotonic dystrophy may occur
in the newborn period, with hypotonia. More
commonly, it presents in the individual's early
second decade of life with limb weakness, distal
wasting, characteristic facies, and cranial muscle
involvement (Fig. 2.38). Learning difficulties may
also be present. Other associated findings include
cataracts, baldness, gonadal atrophy, and glucose
intolerance.

Diagnosis: Diagnosis of myotonic dystrophy is
mainly clinical, although an EMG is characteristic.
A muscle biopsy shows dystrophic changes.

Management: The management of myotonic
dystrophy involves treating the myotonia, although
this treatment does not influence the course of the
disease.

Prognosis: Death from myotonic dystrophy is
usually due to cardiomyopathy or involvement of the
respiratory muscles.

Congenital myotonia   Congenital myotonia, or
Thomsen's disease, is a rare disorder that may be
dominant or recessive. Symptoms include myotonia,
which worsens in cold temperatures and with rest.
Generalized muscle hypertrophy is prominent.

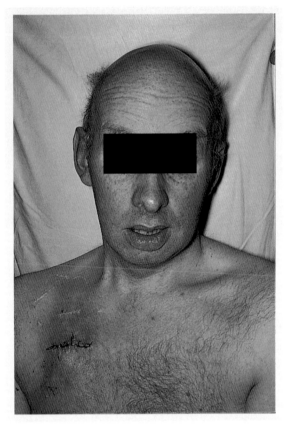

Fig. 2.38 Typical "monk-like" appearance seen in an adult
with myotonic dystrophy. Note the facial weakness,
atrophy of temporal and sternocleidomastoid muscles, and
frontal baldness (courtesy of Dr. GD Perkin).

Paramyotonia congenita   Paramyotonia congenita
is an autosomal dominant condition. The mutation
occurs on chromosome 17, the site coding for the
sodium channel. Paramyotonia congenita is a
nonprogressive muscle weakness that worsens in cold
temperatures.

Metabolic myopathies

The metabolic myopathies are a heterogeneous group
of conditions in which there are abnormalities in
muscle energy metabolism.

Primary metabolic myopathies

Glycogen storage disorders   Glycogen storage
disorders are caused by enzyme anomalies inherited
in a recessive manner. The degree of muscle
involvement is variable between the major types of
primary metabolic myopathies. Symptoms arise as a
result of the decreased availability of energy from

glycolysis because of an impaired ability to mobilize glucose from glycogen.

Glycogen storage disorder type V (McArdle's syndrome) is an autosomal recessive disorder in which there is a deficiency of skeletal muscle myophosphorylase. Symptoms include temporary weakness and muscle cramps on exercise. There is an associated myoglobinuria. There is no rise in venous lactate during exercise, which aids diagnosis by enzyme analysis of muscle tissue. Life expectancy is not affected. Patients are advised to avoid exercise.

Lipid disorders   In the lipid disorders, there is a decreased availability of energy to muscle due to abnormalities in fatty acid metabolism. Patients usually present with hypotonia in infancy or muscle weakness and cramps later in life. Symptoms worsen with prolonged exercise or fasting.

Mitochondrial disorders   The mitochondrial disorders are inherited. These are abnormalities of either the mitochondrial genome (more commonly) or the nuclear genome.

The age of onset is variable. Muscle weakness (particularly of the extraocular muscles) may be isolated or associated with neurologic and metabolic disturbances. Muscle biopsy shows abnormal mitochondria with crystalline inclusions. Mitochondrial myopathy may develop in patients undergoing long-term zidovudine therapy (i.e., patients infected with HIV).

Secondary metabolic myopathies

Myopathic symptoms can occur as a result of a whole range of electrolyte disturbances (e.g., Ca^{2+}, Mg^{2+}, K^+). Endocrine disorders are examples of secondary metabolic myopathies that are acquired.

Periodic paralyses   The periodic paralyses are a rare group of disorders characterized by repeated attacks of muscle weakness. There are three types: hypokalemic, hyperkalemic, and normokalemic.

Hypokalemic periodic paralysis: Hypokalemic periodic paralysis is an autosomal dominant condition. It presents in adolescence and is remitting in a patient's third decade of life.

Attacks often occur after strenuous exercise or a heavy carbohydrate meal. During an attack, the serum potassium concentration is low (2.5–3.5 mmol/L); attacks are terminated by the administration of intravenous potassium chloride. Diuretic therapy and thyrotoxicosis

must be excluded as possible causes of the myopathy.

Hyperkalemic periodic paralysis: Hyperkalemic periodic paralysis is an autosomal dominant condition. It presents in childhood and is remitting in a patient's second decade of life. Attacks may occur after strenuous exercise and are terminated by intravenous calcium gluconate. During an attack, the serum potassium concentration is high (6–7 mmol/L). Attacks last for a shorter period than those associated with hypokalemia.

Normokalemic periodic paralysis: Normokalemic periodic paralysis is a very rare condition. The attacks respond to sodium.

Acquired myopathies
Idiopathic inflammatory myopathies

The idiopathic inflammatory myopathies are uncommon disorders and have a male:female ratio of 1:2. Most people with idiopathic inflammatory myopathy start experiencing symptoms when they reach middle age.

Polymyositis

Polymyositis is the most common inflammatory myopathy.

Etiology: The cause of polymyositis is not known, although it may be autoimmune in origin. A viral cause (coxsackievirus) has been suggested.

Polymyositis is a nonmetastatic complication of malignancy; more than 10% of patients have an underlying malignancy that presents later (e.g., carcinoma of the breast, bronchus, or gastrointestinal tract). In this instance, the male:female ratio is reversed.

Pathology: In polymyositis, inflammation and destruction of both type I and type II muscle fibers occur because of the action of cytotoxic T lymphocytes. Histologically, there is evidence of fiber necrosis, muscle atrophy, and fiber regeneration.

Clinical features: There is progressive, symmetrical, and proximal muscle weakness in a patient with polymyositis. The respiratory and heart muscles may also be affected. Dysphagia and dysarthria are other features.

Polymyositis is associated with other connective tissue diseases, such as SLE and rheumatoid disease. Features typical of connective tissue diseases may be present (e.g., Raynaud's phenomenon, in which there is intermittent vasospasm of arterioles in the hands

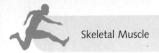

and feet in response to cold and emotional stimuli). It is usually painful, and the affected part of the body goes through the following color changes: pale–blue–red.

Diagnosis: The diagnosis of polymyositis involves two of three findings:

- Raised serum creatine phosphokinase concentrations.
- A characteristic EMG.
- A positive muscle biopsy.

Antinuclear antibodies (Jo–1) and rheumatoid factor may also be present.

Management: The management of polymyositis includes administration of immunosuppressive drugs (causing remission) and physiotherapy to prevent disuse atrophy of muscles. Underlying malignancy must be excluded.

Prognosis: The course of polymyositis is variable. Death results from aspiration pneumonia and respiratory or heart failure.

Dermatomyositis

Dermatomyositis is closely related to polymyositis, sharing features previously described. In addition to muscular symptoms, there are associated skin changes:

- A characteristic purple heliotrope rash, usually on the eyelids, although it may spread to other sites.
- An erythematous rash on the face, scalp, shoulders, and hands.

Inclusion body myositis

Inclusion body myositis affects mainly the elderly and is clinically similar to polymyositis. Electron microscopy demonstrates the presence of filamentous inclusions in the muscle fibers. It is a progressive disorder, and immunosuppressive therapy is not as effective.

Endocrine myopathies (or secondary metabolic myopathies)

Corticosteroid-induced myopathy

Corticosteroid-induced myopathy is caused by an excess of corticosteroid (e.g., as in people with Cushing's syndrome or people on steroid therapy). The myopathy is proximal (i.e., affecting the upper parts of the arms and legs). There is a raised creatine kinase concentration, and muscle biopsy reveals selective atrophy of type II muscle fibers.

Myopathy of thyroid dysfunction

Thyrotoxicosis may be associated with a proximal myopathy. Hypothyroidism may result in symptoms of muscle stiffness and a proximal myopathy.

Myopathy of osteomalacia

All causes of osteomalacia (e.g., vitamin D deficiency, liver failure, liver enzyme-inducing drugs) may result in a proximal myopathy.

 It is useful to remember endocrine and toxic causes of myopathy because they can be easily included on a differential diagnosis list for myopathy.

Toxic myopathies

Toxic myopathies are caused by excessive alcohol intake or drug use.

Excess alcohol   In toxic myopathy caused by excessive alcohol consumption, two patterns of myopathy are seen:

- Subacute proximal myopathy (which may be reversed in the early stages); this is seen in chronic alcoholics. Selective atrophy of type II muscle fibers occurs.
- Acute myopathy associated with severe muscle pain due to acute alcohol excess—myoglobinuria may also occur.

Drug-induced myopathies   Agents that may cause a subacute proximal myopathy include cholesterol-lowering agents (e.g., benzofibrate) as well as chloroquine, penicillamine, and lithium. Patients respond to removal of the drug.

Viral myalgias

The viral myalgias are muscle weaknesses associated with a viral illness, usually respiratory. Myalgic encephalomyelitis (ME, also known as postviral/chronic fatigue syndrome or "yuppie flu") is a disorder in which the patient presents with muscular fatigue and pain on movement. The cause is unknown, and other associated symptoms include poor concentration and depression. The disorder tends to affect women, and opinions differ concerning whether this is a psychological or a musculoskeletal disorder.

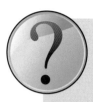

- Outline the differences between the three types of muscle found in the body.
- Identify the sites where the three types of muscle are found.
- Distinguish between neurogenic and myogenic contraction.
- Describe how muscle is arranged and how shape can alter the characteristics of contraction.
- Explain the terms origin, insertion, tendon, aponeurosis, and sesamoid bone.
- Demonstrate diagrammatically the organization of skeletal muscle into fasciculi and muscle fibers.
- Describe the differences between a myofiber, myofibril, and myofilament.
- Explain the term sarcomere.
- Explain the term triad in describing the cellular structure of skeletal muscle.
- Describe the role of satellite cells in adult skeletal muscle.
- Describe the ionic composition of the ICF and ECF in muscle fibers.
- Explain the difference between the RMP and the equilibrium potential.
- Summarize the ionic basis of an AP (e.g., demonstrate on a diagram). Describe its initiation and propagation.
- Explain the following terms: all-or-none law, local circuit theory, and safety factor associated with saltatory conduction.
- With regard to the NMJ, describe the events that occur upon arrival of an AP at the nerve terminal to initiation of an AP in the muscle fiber.
- Describe the synthesis, storage, and breakdown of ACh.
- Explain the types of drugs acting at the NMJ.
- Describe Huxley's cross-bridge cycle and the role of ATP.
- Describe the role of dystrophin protein.
- Explain the terms motor unit, innervation ratio, and size principle.
- Discuss the different types of motor units and relate these to the different muscle fiber types.
- Explain the effects of denervation and reinnervation on motor units.
- Explain the terms isometric and isotonic contraction.
- Describe how summation occurs.
- Identify the difference between tetanus and tetany.
- Draw graphs to demonstrate length–tension and force–velocity relationships.
- Define plasticity.
- Give examples of presynaptic and postsynaptic disorders of the NMJ.
- Explain the pathophysiology, clinical features, and management of myasthenia gravis.
- Describe a simple classification of the inherited myopathies.
- Describe Duchenne muscular dystrophy and give a differential diagnosis.
- Describe the clinical features of myotonic dystrophy.
- Give examples of metabolic myopathies.
- List the three types of periodic paralyses.
- Give a simple classification of the main acquired myopathies.

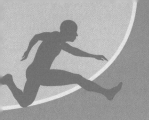

3. Cardiac and Smooth Muscle Types

Cardiac muscle

Structural organization of cardiac muscle

The heart consists of three layers: the inner layer (endocardium), middle layer (myocardium), and outer layer (pericardium) (Fig. 3.1).

Inner layer

The inner layer, or endocardium, is made up of endothelial cells that respond to pressure changes, stretching, and a variety of circulatory substances.

Middle layer

The middle layer, or myocardium, is made up of cardiac muscle cells and is thickest in the ventricles.

Outer layer

The outer layer, or pericardium, consists of three membranes. The two serous membranes are the epicardium (visceral pericardium), which is intimately related to the myocardium, and the parietal pericardium, which lines the inner aspect of the nonserous membrane, the fibrous pericardium. The space between the two serous membranes (visceral and parietal pericardium) is the pericardial cavity. The fibrous pericardium forms the outermost layer of the three membranes.

Microstructure of cardiac muscle

Intercalated discs are low-resistance junctions between myocytes (Fig. 3.2). These allow rapid propagation of action potentials (APs) from cell to cell; hence, the term cardiac syncytium.

Individual skeletal muscle fibers may be regarded as a syncytium because each fiber is made up of a number of myoblasts that have fused. However, skeletal muscle fibers contract independently of each other; therefore, skeletal muscle is not referred to as a syncytium.

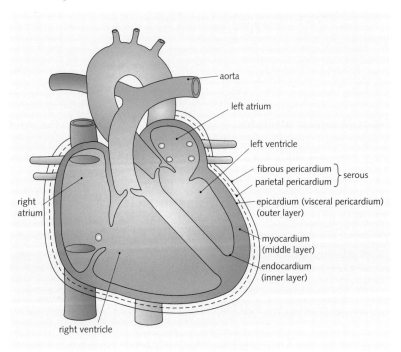

Fig. 3.1 Macroscopic organization of the heart.

- aorta
- left atrium
- left ventricle
- fibrous pericardium
- parietal pericardium } serous
- epicardium (visceral pericardium) (outer layer)
- myocardium (middle layer)
- endocardium (inner layer)
- right atrium
- right ventricle

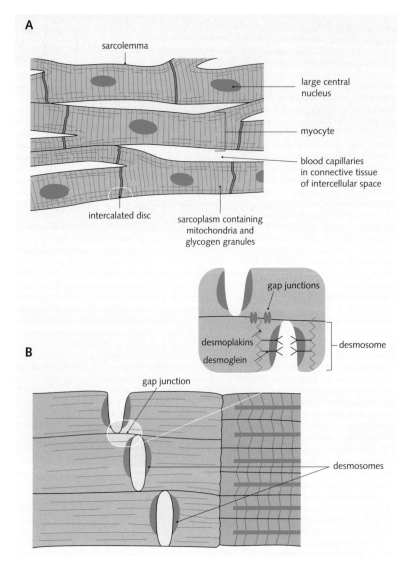

Fig. 3.2 A. Microscopic structure of cardiac muscle. Note that there are far fewer mitochondria in cardiac muscle than in skeletal muscle. B. Components of the intercalated disc.

Types of cardiac myocytes

There are two types of cardiac myocytes (muscle cells): atrial and ventricular. The APs associated with these myocytes vary (Fig. 3.3).

Cellular physiology of cardiac muscle
Initiation of cardiac AP

Under normal circumstances, the AP is initiated in the sinoatrial (SA) node. APs occur at the greatest rate in the SA node; hence, it acts as the pacemaker, setting the rate in other myocytes.

Propagation of cardiac AP

Propagation occurs rapidly, owing to the presence of gap junctions. The AP is propagated from the SA node to the atrioventricular (AV) node. The AP is then propagated to the bundle of His into the left and right bundle branches and Purkinje fibers and into the ventricular myocytes.

Conduction is slow in the AV node, resulting in a delay of 0.1 second before excitation of the ventricles. This delay is important because it results in contraction of the atria before the ventricles, thereby allowing more efficient emptying of the atria.

Ionic basis

There are two types of AP in cardiac muscle.

AP in SA and AV nodes: SA node and AV node cells have the property of automatic

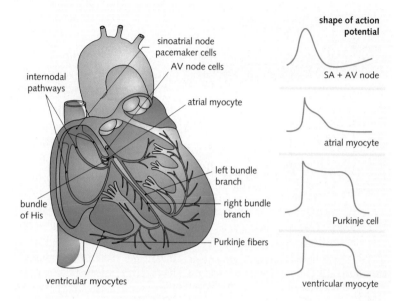

shape of action
potential

SA + AV node

atrial myocyte

Purkinje cell

ventricular myocyte

sinoatrial node
pacemaker cells

AV node cells

atrial myocyte

left bundle
branch

right bundle
branch

Purkinje fibers

internodal
pathways

bundle
of His

ventricular myocytes

Fig. 3.3 Conducting system of the heart showing the location of the different types of myocytes and the action potentials associated with them (AV, atrioventricular; SA, sinoatrial).

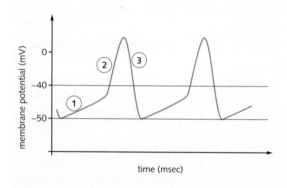

Fig. 3.4 Characteristics of the action potential seen in sinoatrial and atrioventricular node cells. (1) Drifting resting membrane potential caused by slow Na^+ influx, or "pacemaker potential." (2) Influx of Ca^{2+}. (3) Repolarization because of K^+ efflux.

rhythmicity resulting from the leakiness of the membrane to Na^+ in the absence of an AP and a decrease in K^+ conductance. This causes a resting membrane potential (RMP) that drifts from a threshold of -55 mV (lower than the RMP of ventricular and atrial myocytes) to -40 mV. A Ca^{2+} influx is responsible for the rising phase of the AP (Fig. 3.4).

AP in Purkinje cells and *atrial and ventricular myocytes:* Three types of channel are involved in the

AP: fast Na^+ channels, slow Ca^{2+}/Na^+ channels (which are not found in skeletal muscle and are responsible for the plateau phase), and K^+ channels (Fig. 3.5).

The AP in ventricular cells differs from Purkinje cells in that the RMP is level in ventricular myocytes; in Purkinje cells, the RMP slowly rises to threshold (i.e., the cells are self-excitable).

Pacemaker tissue

Under normal conditions, the SA node functions as the heart's pacemaker. In SA node pacemaker cells, APs are generated at a greater rate than in pacemaker tissue elsewhere in the heart. Hence, the SA node sets the rhythm for the heart overall.

Pacemaker tissue is also found in the AV node, bundle of His, and Purkinje fibers. These are often referred to as latent pacemakers because they can take over if the normal pacemaker fails.

Excitation–contraction coupling

Excitation–contraction coupling of cardiac muscle is essentially the same as skeletal muscle. This involves:
- Spread of the AP over the myocyte membrane.
- Influx of Ca^{2+}.
- Contraction due to formation of cross-bridges and sliding of filaments.

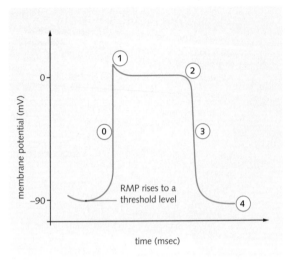

Fig. 3.5 Phases of the cardiac action potential in Purkinje cells. (0) Depolarization because of rapid Na^+ influx. (1) Initial rapid repolarization due to inactivation of Na^+ channels and a passive influx of Cl^-. (2) Prolonged plateau phase with opening of slow Ca^{2+}/Na^+ channels. This prolongs depolarization owing to a Ca^{2+} influx and results in contraction of the myocyte. (3) Late repolarization caused by closure of Ca^{2+}/Na^+ channels and K^+ efflux owing to the opening of K^+ channels. (4) Restoration of RMP (RMP, resting membrane potential).

Bioenergetics of cardiac contraction
Cardiac muscle is mainly dependent on oxidative phosphorylation for contraction because totally anaerobic conditions would not provide sufficient energy to sustain ventricular contraction.

Energy substrates vary according to dietary intake. For example, during starvation, fat is the main substrate. Cardiac muscle has a rich blood supply derived from the coronary arteries during diastole. Cardiac muscle differs from skeletal muscle in that:
- The cardiac AP is 100 times longer.
- There is a long refractory period in cardiac muscle, and, therefore, tetanus does not occur. However, when the frequency of APs is increased, there is an increase in intracellular Ca^{2+} levels. This results in an increase in the force of successive contractions and is known as the treppe or staircase effect.
- Cardiac muscle is self-excitatory.
- The sarcoplasmic reticulum and T tubules are organized in dyads (at the Z lines), not in triads. The sarcoplasmic reticulum is not as well developed and therefore stores less Ca^{2+}. In addition, extracellular Ca^{2+} enters the cell directly through the tubules via slow Ca^{2+} channels. Hence, the force of contraction in cardiac muscle

is largely dependent on the extracellular Ca^{2+} concentration.

Inotropes
Inotropes are agents that increase the force of cardiac contraction (Fig. 3.6).

Mechanism of action
Inotropes increase the intracellular Ca^{2+} concentration. Digitalis glycosides (e.g., digoxin) inhibit the Na^+/K^+ ATPase pump. This results in an increase in intracellular Na^+ and therefore an increase in intracellular Ca^{2+} caused by the action of the Ca^{2+}/Na^+ exchanger.

Sympathomimetics (e.g., dobutamine) act on β_1 receptors, which increase intracellular Ca^{2+} via a rise in cyclic adenosine–5-monophosphate C (cAMP). Phosphodiesterase (PDE) inhibitors (e.g., milrinone) also increase cAMP.

Function of cardiac muscle
Control of heart rate
Heart rate is affected by the autonomic nervous system.

Activation of the parasympathetic (vagal) nerves
Activation of the parasympathetic (vagal) nerves has the effect of decreasing heart rate, decreasing contractility, and slowing transmission of the cardiac impulse. These nerves mainly innervate the SA and AV nodes.

Mechanism of action
Activation of the parasympathetic (vagal) nerves causes hyperpolarization of the myocytic membrane via muscarinic acetylcholine (ACh) receptors. Anticholinergic drugs antagonize this effect.

Activation of the sympathetic system
Activation of the sympathetic system has the effect of increasing heart rate and force of contractility; β-adrenoceptor antagonists inhibit this effect.

Length–tension relationship in cardiac muscle
As with skeletal muscle, the force of contraction increases with muscle fiber length in cardiac muscle.

Starling's law
Starling's law states that the force of contraction is proportional to the initial length of the cardiac muscle fiber. Muscle fiber length increases as the volume of blood in the heart chamber increases.

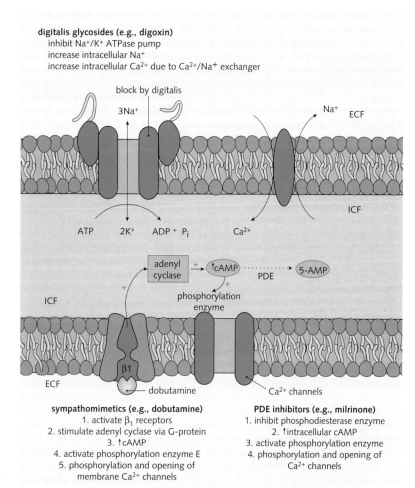

digitalis glycosides (e.g., digoxin)
inhibit Na$^+$/K$^+$ ATPase pump
increase intracellular Na$^+$
increase intracellular Ca^{2+} due to Ca^{2+}/Na$^+$ exchanger

block by digitalis

3Na$^+$

Na$^+$ ECF

ATP   2K$^+$ ADP + P$_i$ Ca^{2+}

ICF

adenyl cyclase + ↑cAMP ------ ► 5-AMP
PDE

ICF   +
phosphorylation enzyme

ECF

β1

dobutamine   Ca^{2+} channels

sympathomimetics (e.g., dobutamine)
1. activate β$_1$ receptors
2. stimulate adenyl cyclase via G-protein
3. ↑cAMP
4. activate phosphorylation enzyme E
5. phosphorylation and opening of
membrane Ca^{2+} channels

PDE inhibitors (e.g., milrinone)
1. inhibit phosphodiesterase enzyme
2. ↑intracellular cAMP
3. activate phosphorylation enzyme
4. phosphorylation and opening of
Ca^{2+} channels

Fig. 3.6 Inotropic drugs and their sites of action in the cardiac cell (PDE, phosphodiesterase; ECF, extracellular fluid; ICF, intracellular fluid).

Within physiologic limits, the heart is able to pump out all the blood entering it. Starling's law does not hold in situations where excessive stretching of cardiac muscle fibers is caused by a decrease in the actin–myosin interaction.

Smooth muscle

The majority of smooth muscle found in the body is of the single-unit type (Fig. 3.7). Examples of multiunit smooth muscle found in the body are the iris and ciliary muscle of the eye.

Organization of smooth muscle
Microstructure of smooth muscle
Smooth muscle cells are spindle-shaped (fusiform) cells that are uninucleate and organized into bundles; sheets; or long, cylindrical units (Fig. 3.8). These are

surrounded by connective tissue containing the nerves and blood vessels.

The cells in a unit are:
• Surrounded by an external lamina.
• Arranged in parallel to one another.
• Offset to each other so the thick middle portion of one is juxtaposed to the thin ends of adjacent cells.
• Adherent at multiple sites.
• Able to communicate with each other via gap junctions (nexus junctions) that are present at sites where the external lamina is deficient.
• Able to contract together as a functional single unit.

Arrangement of smooth muscle in different tissues
Smooth muscle cells are arranged circumferentially in blood vessels and airways (see Fig. 3.8). In

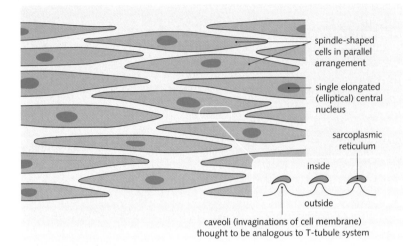

caveoli (invaginations of cell membrane) thought to be analogous to T-tubule system

Fig. 3.7 Microstructure of single-unit (visceral) smooth muscle in longitudinal section.

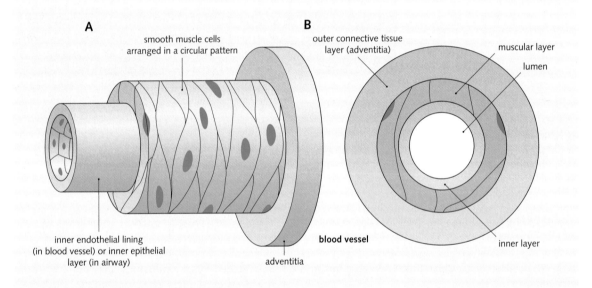

Fig. 3.8 Circumferential arrangement of smooth muscle cells. A. Longitudinal arrangement. B. Transverse arrangement.

the intestines and lower two thirds of the esophagus (the upper third comprises skeletal muscle), smooth muscle is arranged in two layers (Fig. 3.9).

In the inner layer, cells are arranged circumferentially and alter the diameter of the lumen; in the outer layer, cells are arranged longitudinally and influence the length. Both the diameter and length of the tract can be altered, causing movement of contents by peristalsis.

In the stomach, smooth muscle cells are arranged in three layers. These are the:
- Inner oblique layer.
- Middle circular layer.
- Outer longitudinal layer.

In the bladder, smooth muscle cells are arranged in three layers. These are the:
- Inner longitudinal layer.
- Middle circular layer.
- Outer longitudinal layer.

50

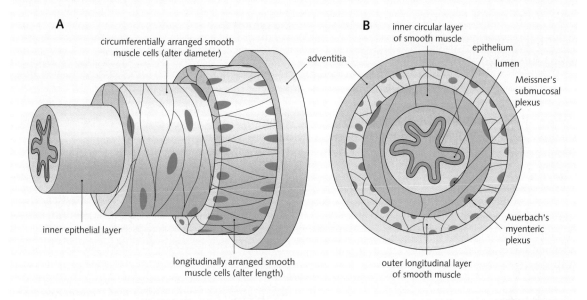

Fig. 3.9 Arrangement of smooth muscle cells in the intestine. A. Longitudinal arrangement. B. Transverse arrangement.

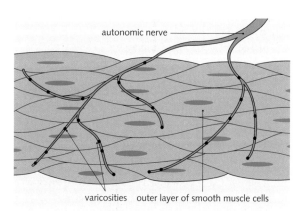

Fig. 3.10 Arrangement of autonomic nerve fibers in smooth muscle.

Cellular physiology of smooth muscle

Initiation of contraction of smooth muscle may result from several mechanisms.

Autonomic nervous system stimulation

In smooth muscle, branching nerve fibers contain neurotransmitter in swellings called varicosities. Released neurotransmitter diffuses to receptors on smooth muscle fiber, so there is usually no direct contact between nerve fibers and muscle cells (Fig. 3.10).

According to the type of receptor activated, the effect will be either excitatory or inhibitory. The neurotransmitter released by a parasympathetic nerve may be ACh or, if released by a sympathetic nerve, noradrenaline. The two types of neurotransmitter have opposite effects in any one tissue.

If a section of smooth muscle has many layers, usually only the outer one is innervated. The resulting AP is conducted to other layers via gap junctions. In the intestinal tract, peristalsis is coordinated by the Auerbach's (myenteric) and Meissner's (submucosal) plexuses that lie on either side of the inner circular layer of smooth muscle closest to the epithelium.

Action of circulating hormones

The most common hormones influencing smooth muscle contraction are ACh, adrenaline, noradrenaline, angiotensin, and vasopressin; others include serotonin and histamine.

These hormones act on receptors on the muscle fiber membrane, resulting in opening/closing of ion channels, thereby initiating or inhibiting APs, and changes in the cell due to activation of second-messenger pathways (e.g., release of Ca^{2+} from the sarcoplasmic reticulum).

A hormone may have an excitatory effect in one tissue type yet an inhibitory effect in

51

another. The type of effect depends on the receptor activated.

Local tissue factors

Local tissue factors involved in smooth muscle tone are CO_2, H^+, and Ca^{2+} (Fig. 3.11). The mechanism by which these produce a contraction is unclear.

Contractile apparatus

Smooth muscle has three types of contractile protein: actin, myosin, and desmin (Fig. 3.12). Desmin is an intermediate filament.

The proteins criss-cross the cell and are anchored at cytoskeletal points called focal densities or dense bodies (analogous to Z discs in skeletal muscle). Focal densities transmit the force of contraction to surrounding smooth muscle cells. This allows smooth muscle cells to contract as one unit.

Smooth muscle AP

In smooth muscle, the RMP is usually about -50 to -60 mV (i.e., less negative than skeletal muscle), and Ca^{2+}, not Na^+, is usually responsible for the AP. The AP can be spike-like (skeletal muscle) or plateau-like. Smooth muscle cells communicate electrically via gap (nexus) junctions.

Excitation–contraction coupling

During excitation–contraction coupling of smooth muscle, there is a rise in intracellular Ca^{2+}. Four Ca^{2+} bind to calmodulin protein present in the cytoplasm. This results in the formation of a myosin kinase–calmodulin–Ca^{2+} complex.

Myosin kinase phosphorylates a site on the myosin light chain. The phosphorylated myosin is then able to interact with actin to form cross-bridges. A decrease in myoplasmic Ca^{2+} concentration inactivates myosin kinase—the enzyme is only active when it is part of the calmodulin complex. The dephosphorylation of myosin takes place by myosin phosphatase.

Regulation of intracellular Ca^{2+} concentration

In smooth muscle, intracellular Ca^{2+} is elevated by:
- Mobilization of intracellular stores: Ca^{2+} is rapidly released from the sarcoplasmic reticulum upon activation of the cell.
- Voltage-activated Ca^{2+} channels in the sarcolemma.
- Receptor-activated Ca^{2+} channels in the sarcolemma.
- Caveoli—invaginations in the sarcolemma believed to be analogous to T tubules in skeletal muscle. The exact mechanism by which they control the entry of Ca^{2+} into the cell is unknown.

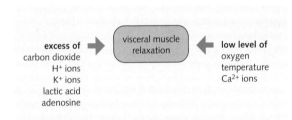

Fig. 3.11 Effect of local tissue factors on the tone of smooth muscle.

Intracellular Ca^{2+} concentration is restored by:
- Active pumping back into the sarcoplasmic reticulum.
- Active pumping of Ca^{2+} out of the cell.
- Na^+/Ca^{2+} exchange across the sarcolemma.

Smooth muscle contraction differs from skeletal muscle in that troponin is not a component of the thin filament, and Ca^{2+} binds to the cytoplasmic protein calmodulin.

Disadvantages of smooth muscle contraction are that:
- Phosphorylation is a relatively slow process; therefore, cross-bridge turnover and contraction velocities are low.
- Adenosine triphosphate (ATP) is required for both phosphorylation and powering of cross-bridges. Therefore, smooth muscle contraction is less efficient.

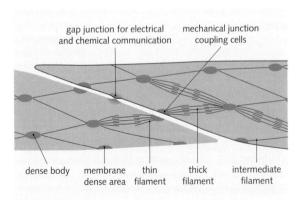

Fig. 3.12 Organization of contractile proteins in smooth muscle (adapted from *Physiology*, 3rd ed., by Berne RM and Levy MN, Mosby Year Book, 1993).

Advantages of slow cross-bridge turnover are that:
- The lower ATP consumption is adequately provided by oxidative phosphorylation; hence, no fatigue is shown.
- There is prolonged contraction.

Organic nitrates

Examples of organic nitrates include glyceryl trinitrate and isosorbide dinitrate.

Mechanism of action: Organic nitrates relax smooth muscle by increasing intracellular nitric oxide (NO) that interferes with contractile proteins and Ca^{2+} regulation.

Indications: Organic nitrates are drugs used in the treatment of angina and hypertension.

Adverse effects: There are no serious side effects from organic nitrates, although headache and postural hypotension may occur.

The organic nitrates act in the same way as the vasodilator NO produced by endothelial cells. Prostacyclin is also a vasodilator produced by endothelial cells. The vasoconstrictor released by endothelial cells is endothelin.

Functions of smooth muscle

The functions of smooth muscle depend on the site:
- In blood vessels and airways, smooth muscle is important in maintaining tone and diameter.
- In the gastrointestinal tract, it is important in mixing and propelling the contents along the tract via peristalsis.
- In the urinary system, the muscle is responsible for propelling urine and emptying the bladder.

Myoepithelial cells

Myoepithelial cells are contractile cells found in mammary glands, sweat glands, salivary glands, and the iris. They contain a layer of flat cells arranged around acini and ducts. The arrangement of contractile proteins is similar to that in smooth muscle. Upon stimulation, myoepithelial cells contract and cause expulsion of glandular secretions or changes in the aperture of the pupil.

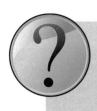

- Explain the term cardiac syncytium.
- Describe the initiation and propagation of the cardiac AP.
- Describe the ionic basis of the AP in the SA node compared to that in the Purkinje cells.
- Describe the differences in contraction of cardiac muscle to that in skeletal muscle.
- Explain the effect of the autonomic nervous system on heart rate.
- Describe how smooth muscle cells are arranged.
- Illustrate the arrangement of myofilaments in smooth muscle.
- Describe the mechanisms involved in changing intracellular calcium levels.
- Describe how smooth muscle contraction differs from skeletal muscle contraction and the effect of this difference.
- Outline the functions of smooth muscle in the body.
- What is the treppe or staircase effect?

4. Bone

Overview of the skeleton

The skeletal system is composed of various types of connective tissue, including bone and cartilage. Bone and cartilage contain cells embedded in an extracellular matrix. This matrix consists of an amorphous ground substance permeated by a system of collagen and elastic fibers. These fibers differ from general connective tissue because their matrices are solid; however, they do share the same origin from embryonic cellular connective tissue, the mesenchyme.

Components of the skeleton
Bone
Bone is rigid and forms most of the skeleton. It is the main supporting tissue of the body and provides a framework for most of the body's tissues.

Cartilage
Cartilage is a resilient tissue that provides semirigid support for certain parts of the skeleton (e.g., the costal cartilages, respiratory airways, and external ear).

Joints
Joints are composite structures that unite the bones of the skeleton. Depending on their form, joints allow for varying degrees of movement and stability of the skeleton.

Ligaments and tendons
Ligaments and tendons are fibrous tissues that form part of the musculoskeletal system. Ligaments are flexible bands that connect bone or cartilage, thus stabilizing and strengthening joints. Tendons are the connections between muscles and their points of insertion into bones.

Functions of the skeleton
The skeleton performs the following functions:
- Offers support for the body because it is a rigid framework.
- Protects the organs (e.g., the neurocranium around the brain and the thoracic cage around the heart and lungs).
- Provides a mechanical basis for locomotion.
- Offers mineral storage—the majority of calcium, phosphorus, and magnesium salts are found in bone.
- Provides the site for bone marrow, where the development of blood cells, or hematopoiesis, occurs postnatally.

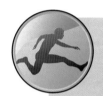

In newborn infants, red bone marrow produces red blood cells, some lymphocytes, granulocytic white blood cells, and platelets. In adults, yellow bone marrow is mature bone marrow that has filled with adipocytes.

Organization of bone and cartilage

Distribution of bone and cartilage
The human skeleton is bilaterally symmetrical. It comprises the axial and appendicular skeleton (Fig. 4.1).

The axial skeleton consists of the bones of the head (skull), neck (hyoid bone and cervical vertebrae), and trunk (ribs, sternum, thoracic and lumbar vertebrae, and sacrum).

The appendicular skeleton consists of the bones of the upper and lower limbs and includes those forming the pectoral and pelvic girdles.

With increasing age, the proportions of bone and cartilage in the skeleton change. In the fetus, most long bones are initially represented by hyaline cartilage that resembles the shape of adult bone. In the adult, the only remnants of hyaline cartilage are the articular cartilages of joints, the tracheal rings, the skeleton of the larynx, the cartilages of the nasal skeleton, and the anterior aspects of the ribs.

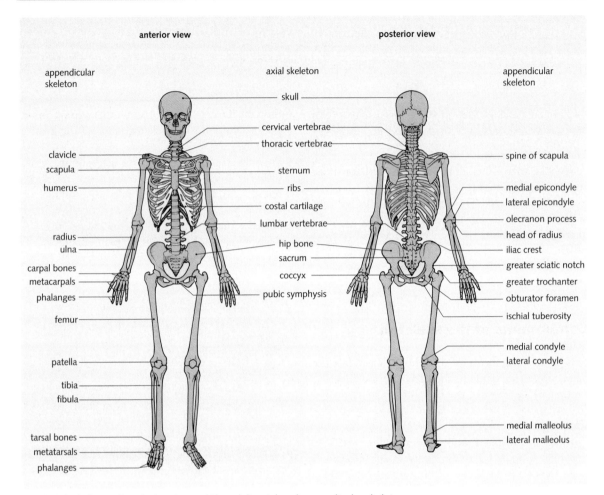

anterior view   posterior view

appendicular   axial skeleton   appendicular
skeleton   skeleton

skull

cervical vertebrae
thoracic vertebrae

clavicle   spine of scapula
scapula
humerus   sternum   medial epicondyle
                                ribs   lateral epicondyle
                                costal cartilage   olecranon process
                                lumbar vertebrae   head of radius

radius   hip bone   iliac crest
ulna   sacrum   greater sciatic notch
carpal bones   coccyx   greater trochanter
metacarpals   obturator foramen
phalanges   pubic symphysis   ischial tuberosity

femur
                                                                  medial condyle
                                                                  lateral condyle
patella

tibia
fibula

                                                                  medial malleolus
                                                                  lateral malleolus

tarsal bones
metatarsals
phalanges

Fig. 4.1 Anterior and posterior views of the adult axial and appendicular skeleton.

Cartilage
Cartilage microstructure
Cartilage consists of cells called chondroblasts and chondrocytes that are embedded within an extensive matrix. This matrix is composed of fibrous elements and a ground substance. The chondroblasts and chondrocytes produce and maintain the matrix.

Cartilage formation and cell types
Cartilage derives from mesenchyme, embryonic cellular connective tissue. During development, the primitive mesenchymal cells become round, retract their extensions, and undergo rapid mitotic divisions. This process forms mesenchymal condensations.

Chondroblasts
Chondroblasts are the precursors of cartilage and arise from the differentiation of mesenchyme. They secrete cartilage matrix. The synthesis and deposition of this matrix separates the chondroblasts from each other and traps them within the matrix. Each chondroblast then undergoes up to eight further mitotic divisions to form groups of isogenous cells (i.e., developed from the same cell) surrounded by a smaller amount of condensed matrix.

Chondrocytes
Chondrocytes are mature cartilage cells occupying small cavities, or lacunae, in the matrix. Chondrocytes maintain the integrity of the matrix. Chondrocytes that are active have a basophilic

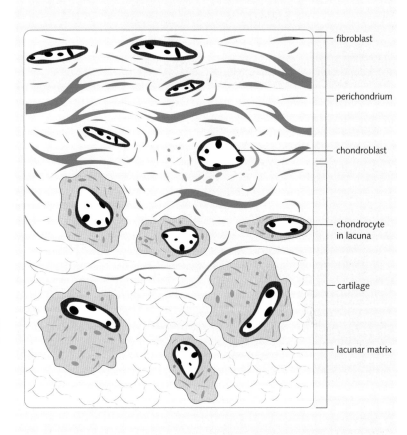

fibroblast

perichondrium

chondroblast

chondrocyte in lacuna

cartilage

lacunar matrix

Fig. 4.2 Diagram of an area of perichondrium overlying hyaline cartilage. Perichondrial cells differentiate into chondroblasts and then chondrocytes, growing in from the periphery. Cartilage matrix lies between the cells; it is rich in collagen, apart from the lacunae that are rich in glycosaminoglycans (adapted from *Basic Histology*, 8th ed., by Junqueira LC, Appleton & Lange, 1995).

cytoplasm (indicating protein synthesis), plenty of rough endoplasmic reticulum, and a large Golgi complex. Older, less active cells are smaller and have a pale cytoplasm and reduced Golgi complex.

The sequence of differentiation and maturation of cartilage cells is most developed in the center of growing cartilage. Toward the periphery of the cartilage, chondroblasts at earlier stages of maturation merge with the surrounding perichondrium (Fig. 4.2).

Perichondrial cells differentiate into chondroblasts and then into chondrocytes, growing inward from the periphery. Cartilage matrix, which is rich in collagen, lies between the cells. The lacunae are rich in glycosaminoglycans.

Matrix

Cartilage matrix is firm and solid but pliable, causing it to be resilient. The matrix contains varying types and amounts of fibers and ground substance. The fibers are made up of either collagen—type II (hyaline) and type I (fibrocartilage)—or elastin.

The ground substance is rich in glycosaminoglycans. Chondroitin and keratin sulfates are joined to a core protein to form a proteoglycan monomer. A hyaluronic acid molecule is associated with about 80 proteoglycan units; these are joined by link proteins to form a large hyaluronate proteoglycan aggregate. Cross-linking glycoproteins bind these aggregates to collagen fibrils in the tissue (Fig. 4.3).

Perichondrium

All hyaline cartilage, apart from articular cartilage, is covered by a layer of perichondrium. This is a dense connective tissue. Perichondrium is rich in type I collagen fibers. The outer layer contains fibroblasts, and the inner layer has chondroblasts.

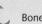
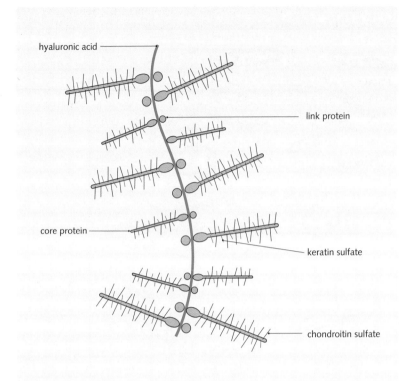

Fig. 4.3 Proteoglycan macromolecule formed from chondroitin and keratin sulfates joined to a core protein.

Growth

Cartilage can increase in size by either interstitial growth or appositional growth.

Interstitial growth

Interstitial growth takes place in the middle of cartilage by the mitotic division of mature chondrocytes. This growth occurs in relatively young cartilage, which is malleable enough to allow for internal expansion.

Appositional growth

Appositional growth occurs on the periphery of cartilage from the differentiation of perichondrial cells.

Blood supply

Because mature cartilage is an avascular tissue, the exchange of metabolites between chondrocytes and surrounding tissue relies on diffusion through the matrix. In sites where cartilage is particularly thick (e.g., costal cartilage), small blood vessels are carried into the center of the tissue by cartilage canals. Poor blood supply to cartilage:

- Limits the extent of its thickness, because the innermost cells need to be maintained.
- Makes repair after injury difficult, because injured areas are usually replaced by fibrous tissue.

Cartilage types

Cartilage type depends on the composition of its matrix components. Three types of cartilage occur: hyaline cartilage, elastic cartilage, and fibrocartilage.

Hyaline cartilage

Hyaline cartilage is the most common type of cartilage. It is characterized by a uniformly amorphous matrix and contains type II collagen fibers oriented along lines of stress.

Throughout childhood and adolescence, hyaline cartilage is present in the epiphyseal plates of long bones. It has a great resistance to wear and a very low coefficient of friction, and it covers the surface of nearly all synovial joints, or areas that are subjected to a great deal of stress.

Elastic cartilage

Elastic cartilage is composed of large numbers of elastic fibers and elastic lamellae embedded in matrix, which make the cartilage flexible. It is found in the auricle of the ear, the external auditory meatus, the auditory tube, parts of the larynx, and the epiglottis.

Fibrocartilage
Fibrocartilage comprises a large number of type I collagen fibers embedded in a small amount of matrix. It is found in discs within joints (e.g., the intervertebral, temporomandibular, sternoclavicular, and knee joints) and also on the articular surfaces of the clavicle and the mandible.

Bone
Bone shape
Bone is described according to its shape: long, short, flat, irregular, or sesamoid.

Long bones
Long bones are longer than its width; most bone in the appendicular skeleton is of this type. The ends of long bones are composed of cancellous (spongy, trabecular) bone surrounded by a thin layer of compact bone. Their shafts contain a bony network along stress-bearing lines and surround cavities filled with bone marrow. The articular surfaces are covered by hyaline (articular) cartilage.

Short bones
Short bones have a length and width of similar size and is roughly cuboidal or round in shape. Such bones are found in the wrist and ankle. Short bone is composed of cancellous bone surrounded by a thin layer of compact bone and is covered by periosteum. Hyaline cartilage covers the articulating surfaces.

Flat bones
Flat bones are usually thin, flat, and curved. They are found in the vault of the skull (calveria), ribs, sternum, and scapulae. It consists of thin inner and outer layers of compact bone separated by a layer of cancellous bone called the diploë.

Irregular bones
Irregular bones do not fit into any of the previous groups. Vertebrae and sphenoid bone are examples of this type. Irregular bone is composed of cancellous bone with a covering of thin compact bone.

Sesamoid bones
Sesamoid bones are small bones found in some tendons, such as those that rub over bony surfaces. Tendons such as the quadriceps femoris and flexor pollicis brevis contain the patella and the sesamoid bones, respectively. Most of a sesamoid bone is buried in the tendon; the free surface is covered with cartilage. Sesamoid bone reduces friction on the tendon and may also alter its direction of pull.

Bone anatomy
Long bones
Long bones have a shaft called the diaphysis; each end is expanded into an epiphysis (Fig. 4.4).

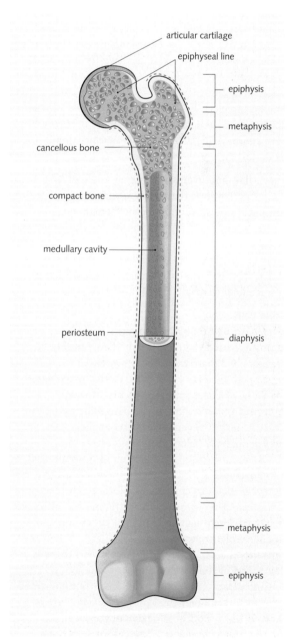

Fig. 4.4 Features of long bone.

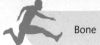

The diaphysis contains a large central medullary cavity surrounded by a thick-walled tube of compact bone. A small amount of cancellous bone lines the inner surface of the compact bone, forming a network of trabeculae.

In adults, the medullary cavity is filled with yellow (inactive) marrow, which is mostly adipose tissue; red (active) marrow is confined to the proximal epiphyses of larger adult long bone. The epiphyses consist mainly of cancellous bone and have a thin outer shell of compact bone. Their articular surfaces are covered with a layer of hyaline cartilage.

In growing bone, the site of elongation of the bone is known as the epiphyseal cartilage (growth plate). When bone stops growing, the epiphyseal growth plate becomes ossified and forms the epiphyseal line. The metaphysis, the flared epiphyseal end of the diaphyses, is very vascular. Long bone is covered by periosteum (except the articular surfaces) and lined by endosteum.

Short, flat, and irregular bone
Bone that is short, flat, and irregular is composed of compact bone surrounding cancellous bone.

Bone microstructure
Bone is composed of cells called osteoblasts, osteocytes, and osteoclasts that are embedded in an extracellular matrix.

Bone cells
Osteoblasts: Osteoblasts lie on the inner layer of the periosteum and the endosteum. They secrete an organic bone matrix in which they become entrapped, forming osteocytes. Active osteoblasts have a large Golgi complex, plenty of rough endoplasmic reticulum, and a basophilic cytoplasm. Resting (inactive) osteoblasts are smaller, flattened cells and have a paler cytoplasm.

Osteocytes: Osteocytes are found in small cavities called lacunae. Each cell has many processes that run along canaliculi to connect with other cells via gap junctions. Osteocytes maintain the matrix, although they have less rough endoplasmic reticulum and a smaller Golgi complex than osteoblasts. When the cells die, the lacunae remain empty, and there is resorption of the matrix.

Osteoclasts: Osteoclasts are large multinucleated cells with many branched processes. They are derived from the fusion of monocytes in blood and are therefore phagocytic. The cells resorb bone and are found in troughs, called Howship's lacunae,

and on surfaces where bone is being removed. Cells in the process of actively resorbing have a pale acidophilic cytoplasm and have many vacuoles and lysosomes for enzymatic digestion. They also have a ruffled border facing the bone matrix; an adjacent clear zone is responsible for adhesion to the matrix and provides a suitable environment of low pH for the lysosomal enzymes.

Bone matrix
Bone matrix has an organic component, which is responsible for flexible strength, and an inorganic component, which is responsible for rigidity and mechanical strength.

The organic matrix (osteoid) is composed of type I collagen embedded in a ground substance of proteoglycan aggregates. Also present are specific glycoproteins, such as bone sialoprotein (rich in sialic acid) and osteocalcin (binds calcium).

The inorganic matrix is composed of deposited mineral salts that make up more than half the weight of dried matrix. The most abundant minerals in the inorganic matrix are calcium and phosphate. These form hydroxyapatite crystals $[Ca_{10}(PO_4)_6(OH)_2]$, the surface ions of which are hydrated to facilitate the exchange of water between the mineral crystals and body fluids. Bicarbonate, citrate, potassium, and sodium are also found but in smaller quantities.

Periosteum
Periosteum covers the outer surface of bone, except articular surfaces. Its outer layer contains blood vessels, nerves, and lymphatics, and its inner layer has a few osteoblasts and osteoclasts.

Sharpey's fibers penetrate into the outer layer of bone to hold the periosteum, ligaments, and tendons in place. Rheumatoid arthritis commonly begins at the sites of insertion of ligaments and tendons into bone.

Endosteum
Endosteum is a single layer of tissue containing osteoblasts and osteoclasts. It lines inner bone surfaces.

Blood supply and lymph drainage of bone
Several arteries supply blood to bone; they enter the bone from the periosteum (Fig. 4.5). These blood vessels include:
- The periosteal arteries, which enter the bone shaft at many points and supply the compact bone. Near the midshaft of the bone, a nutrient artery passes

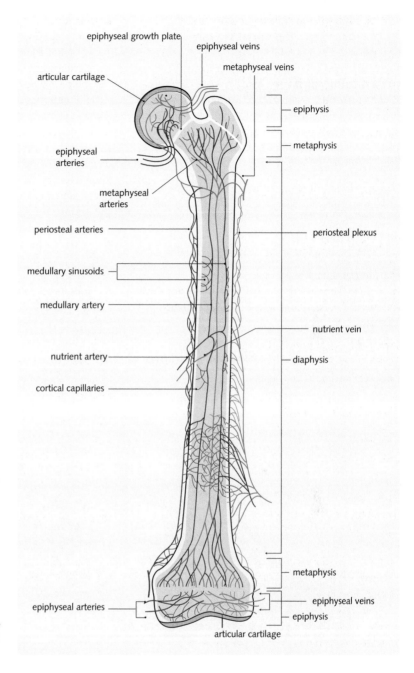

Fig. 4.5 Blood supply of bone. The periosteal, epiphyseal, and nutrient arteries supply the bone.

The labels in the figure are:
epiphyseal growth plate
epiphyseal veins
metaphyseal veins
articular cartilage
epiphysis
metaphysis
epiphyseal arteries
metaphyseal arteries
periosteal arteries
periosteal plexus
medullary sinusoids
medullary artery
nutrient vein
nutrient artery
diaphysis
cortical capillaries
metaphysis
epiphyseal arteries
epiphyseal veins
epiphysis
articular cartilage

through the compact bone to supply the cancellous bone and bone marrow.

• The metaphyseal and epiphyseal arteries, which supply the ends of the bone.

The arteries are accompanied by veins. They are large and numerous in long bone and in areas of red bone marrow. The veins exit through vascular foramina near the articular ends of bones. Lymph vessels are most abundant in the periosteum. They drain into the regional lymph nodes.

Nerve supply of bone
Many nerve fibers travel with the blood vessels to bone. They are mostly vasomotor, meaning they cause constriction or dilatation of blood

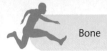
vessels. Periosteal nerves are sensory and contain pain fibers. They are very sensitive to tearing or tension.

Classification of bone

Two types of bone exist: immature or woven bone and mature or lamellar bone. The type of bone is determined by the pattern of collagen deposited.

Immature (woven) bone

In immature (woven) bone, an irregular array of coarse collagen fibers, a large number of osteocytes, and a low mineral content make it mechanically weak. Immature bone is the first type of bone to develop in the embryo and after fractures; it is gradually remodeled and replaced by lamellar bone.

Mature (lamellar) bone

In mature (lamellar) bone, collagen fibers appear in a regular parallel arrangement and have a highly organized infrastructure; these characteristics make the bone mechanically strong (Fig. 4.6).

Lamellar bone may be formed either as compact or cancellous bone.

Compact bone: Compact bone is composed of parallel columns along the long axis of a bone. Each column is made of concentric osteocyte layers fixed in the matrix in cavities called lacunae. The lacunae surround central neurovascular channels called haversian canals. The units of lamellae and canals are known as haversian systems or osteons. The vertical haversian canals are linked with each other and with the endosteum and periosteum via transverse Volkmann's canals. Circumferential lamellae cover the outer surface of compact bone. Interstitial lamellae, which are remnants following bone remodeling, are also present.

Cancellous bone: Cancellous bone contains lamellae that form lattices called trabeculae. They

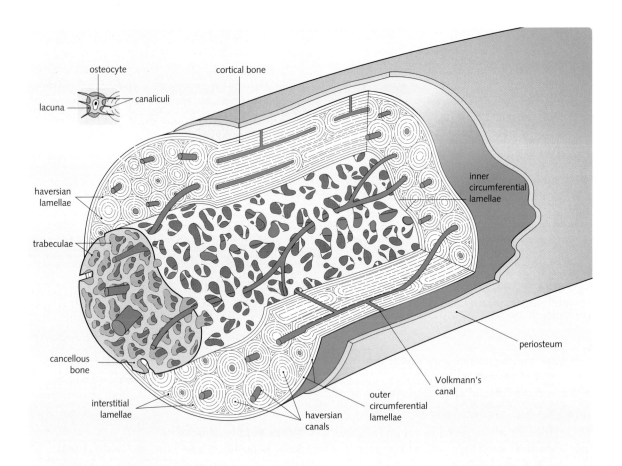

Fig. 4.6 Arrangement of mature bone.

are oriented along lines of stress and provide structural strength. Cancellous bone has greater metabolic activity; hence, it is more affected in conditions such as osteoporosis.

Bone formation, growth, and remodeling

Types of ossification

Although all bones are derived from mesenchyme, the type of process they undergo for their formation, called ossification, can be either intramembranous or endochondral. In intramembranous ossification, bone develops directly from primitive mesenchyme tissue (e.g., the skull bones and clavicle). In endochondral ossification, bone develops indirectly from mesenchyme through an initial cartilage model (i.e., most long bones are formed through endochondral ossification). The two processes result in an identical bone microstructure—both compact and cancellous bone can develop from either method.

After ossification, immature bone grows and is continuously remodeled by osteoclasts and osteoblasts until it is mature. This process continues throughout life. The development of bone is controlled by hormones: growth hormone, thyroid hormones, and sex hormones.

Intramembranous ossification

Intramembranous ossification occurs in "membranes" of condensed mesenchyme tissue. Ossification takes place outward from the center (Fig. 4.7).

Some mesenchymal cells differentiate into osteoblasts at primary ossification centers. Osteoblasts secrete new bone matrix that calcifies and encapsulates the cells in lacunae. These cells then become known as osteocytes. Osteoprogenitor cells beneath the periosteum divide mitotically to produce additional osteoblasts that will lay down more bone. This process forms the outer surface of bone.

Islands of new bone tissue in the mesenchyme are known as spicules. Spicules are penetrated by blood vessels and hematopoietic precursor cells, which will become bone marrow. As bone formation progresses, there is fusion of adjacent centers of ossification to form immature bone with a woven appearance.

Endochondral ossification

Endochondral ossification refers to new bone formation occurring from established cartilage models. Chondroblasts develop in the primitive mesenchyme (Fig. 4.8, A), forming a hyaline cartilage and perichondrium precursor model (Fig. 4.8, B).

Osteoprogenitor cells and osteoblasts are formed at the midshaft of the diaphysis, creating

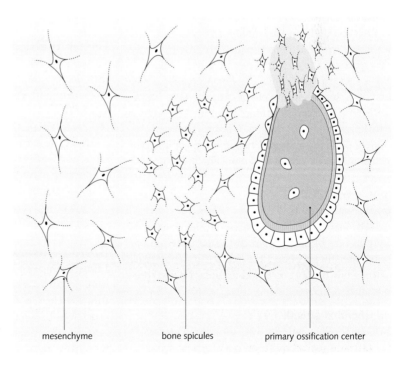

Fig. 4.7 Intramembranous ossification. Some mesenchymal cells differentiate into osteoblasts in the primary ossification center. The islands of bone formed in the mesenchyme that will eventually become bone marrow are known as spicules (adapted from *Basic Histology*, 8th ed., by Junqueira LC, Appleton & Lange, 1995).

mesenchyme   bone spicules   primary ossification center

63

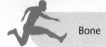

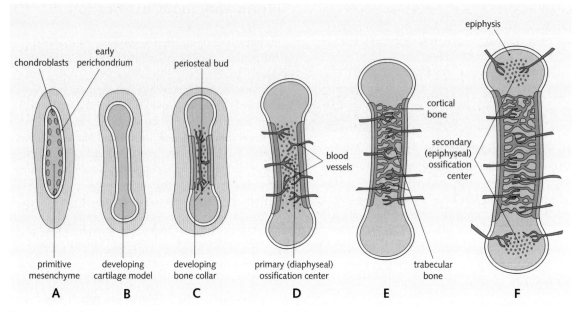

Fig. 4.8 Endochondral ossification. Parts A–F are explained in the text.

periosteum and a collar of bone by intramembranous ossification. Calcium is deposited in the cartilage matrix (Fig. 4.8, C). Blood vessels grow from the periosteum and bone collar. They transport osteoprogenitor cells that differentiate to create a primary ossification center in the middle of the diaphysis (Fig. 4.8, D).

Osteoblasts form lamellae on the calcified cartilage to make lamellar bone. This growth spreads outward from the center. The outer bone collar makes cortical bone. This happens prenatally, when the epiphyses are still made of cartilage (Fig. 4.8, E). Secondary ossification centers form in the epiphyses at different times, mostly after birth. There is endochondral growth until fusion of the epiphyses occurs at around 25 years of age (Fig. 4.8, F).

Bone growth
Appositional growth
Appositional growth involves bone formation on the outer surface of bone to which the periosteum contributes. In long bone, this results in an increase in width, while in short, flat, and irregular bone, there is an increase in general size.

Endochondral growth
Endochondral growth involves interstitial growth of a cartilage model and then replacement with bone (Fig. 4.9). Overall, this results in an increase in bone length.

At the epiphyseal plate, the diaphysis lengthens until the plate becomes fused, forming the epiphyseal line at puberty. At articular cartilage, endochondral growth results in enlargement of the epiphyses.

Factors affecting growth
Factors that have an influence on bone growth include:
- Genetic influences, which determine bone shape and size.
- Dietary factors, such as vitamins D and C, which affect the formation of the organic and inorganic components of bone matrix.
- Hormones, such as growth hormone, thyroid hormones, and sex hormones, usually stimulate bone growth and also cause fusion of the epiphyseal plates to stop bone growth.

Bone remodeling
Immature woven bone undergoes progressive remodeling by osteoclastic resorption and osteoblastic deposition to form mature compact or cancellous bone (Fig. 4.10).

Cancellous bone is laid along fibers of the mesenchyme, and compact bone is laid beneath the

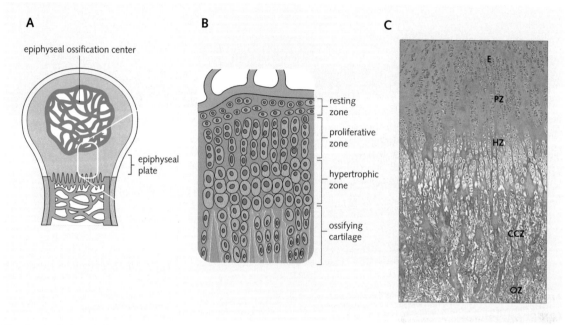

Fig. 4.9 Endochondral growth. A. Epiphyseal ossification center. B. Detail of epiphyseal plate. C. Low-power electron micrograph (E, resting zone of the epiphyseal plate cartilage; PZ, proliferative zone; HZ, hypertrophic zone; CCZ, calcified cartilage zone; OZ, beginning of the ossification zone) (courtesy of Dr. A Stevens and Prof. J Lowe).

periosteum. The primitive mesenchyme that remains in the network of developing bone differentiates into bone marrow.

Functions of bone

Maintenance of calcium levels

Bone, although rigid, is an extremely dynamic tissue. The skeleton contains 99% of the body's calcium. It maintains the levels of calcium in the blood within narrow limits so that muscle contraction and membrane potential activity can occur.

Normally, calcium levels in blood and tissues are stable, and there is a continuous interchange of calcium between the blood and bone (Fig. 4.11).

When levels of calcium in the blood decrease, calcium is mobilized from bones. Conversely, excess levels of calcium in the blood can be removed and stored in bone. One method for regulating blood calcium levels involves the transfer of calcium ions, first from hydroxyapatite crystals to interstitial fluid and then into blood. This takes place in cancellous bone and is a rapid mechanism helped by the large surface area of the hydroxyapatite crystals.

Other ways of regulating blood calcium levels are through parathyroid hormone and calcitonin release (Fig. 4.12). Refer to *Crash Course: Endocrine and Reproductive Systems* for more details about hormones.

Parathyroid hormone

Parathyroid hormone (PTH), also known as parathormone, is a peptide made of 84 amino acids that acts as the main regulator of calcium levels in blood. PTH is secreted from the parathyroid glands in response to low blood calcium levels to raise those levels to normal. When blood calcium levels are high, less PTH is secreted.

PTH stimulates osteoclast activity and results in bone resorption and calcium release into blood. It also increases renal resorption so that less calcium is lost in the urine. PTH also promotes the formation of vitamin D in the kidneys. Vitamin D increases the absorption of calcium from the small intestine.

Hyperparathyroidism, the excessive production of PTH, leads to demineralized bone and elevated blood calcium levels. The excess calcium is deposited at other sites, such as arterial walls and the kidneys.

65

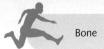

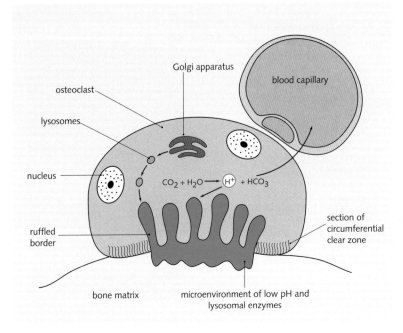

Fig. 4.10 Osteoclastic resorption in bone remodeling (adapted from *Basic Histology*, 8th ed., by Junqueira LC, Appleton & Lange, 1995).

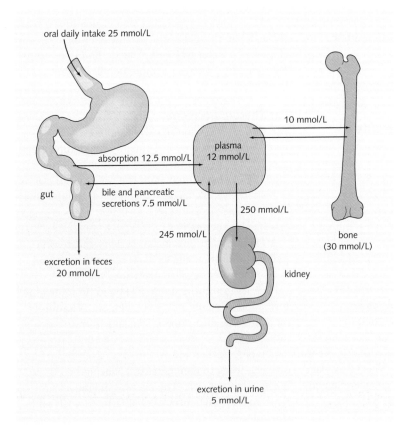

Fig. 4.11 Daily calcium exchange in the body tissues. A continuous exchange of calcium between blood and bone takes place to keep calcium levels stable.

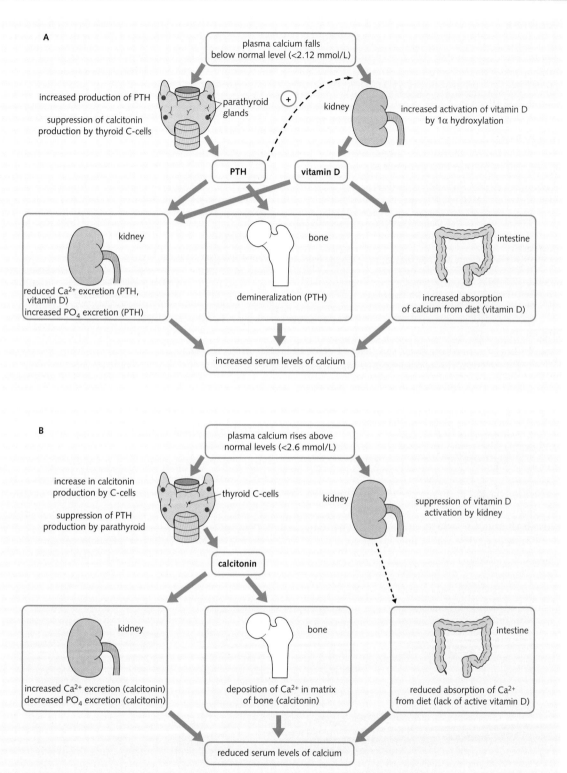

Fig. 4.12 Control of serum calcium levels by parathyroid hormone (PTH), calcitonin, and vitamin D. A. Serum calcium falls below normal levels. B. Serum calcium rises above normal levels.

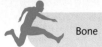

Calcitonin

Calcitonin is responsible for reducing high blood calcium levels to normal. It is a peptide made of 32 amino acids and is secreted from the parafollicular cells of the thyroid gland in response to high blood calcium levels.

Calcitonin inhibits osteoclast activity and opposes the action of PTH. It also decreases calcium and phosphate resorption in the kidney. Excessive calcitonin production has no effect on calcium balance, so people with no calcitonin (e.g., thyroidectomy patients) do not need hormone replacement. The reasons for this are unknown.

Nutrition

During growth, bone is sensitive to nutritional factors. For bone and matrix formation to occur, a person's diet needs to contain proteins, calcium, and vitamins D and C.

Vitamin D

Vitamin D is required for the absorption of calcium and phosphate from the small intestine and, to a lesser extent, the kidney (see Fig. 4.12). It also stimulates calcium resorption from bone. Small amounts of vitamin D occur in foods, such as fish liver oil and egg yolks. Most vitamin D, however, is produced in the epidermis from 7-dehydrocholesterol by a photolytic reaction mediated by ultraviolet light (Fig. 4.13).

Hydroxylation occurs in the endoplasmic reticulum of liver hepatocytes to form 25-hydroxyvitamin D_3, which enters the circulation and is transported to the kidney by vitamin D-binding protein.

Further hydroxylation to 1,25-dihydroxyvitamin D_3 takes place in the mitochondria of the proximal tubules of the kidney. This most active form of vitamin D is called calcitriol. Its synthesis is promoted by PTH, and it has similar actions to PTH.

A decrease in vitamin D can lead to demineralization and poor calcification of bone. This condition is called osteomalacia in adults, but it is called rickets in children because their epiphyseal lines have yet to fuse. Both conditions involve a loss of bone density, a large epiphyses, and bowing of the legs.

Vitamin C

Vitamin C is essential for the synthesis of collagen in the bone matrix by osteoblasts. It is a reducing agent required for the hydroxylation of collagen residues to allow calcification to occur. Vitamin C is found in fresh fruit and vegetables.

A deficiency of vitamin C results in scurvy. The defective connective tissue leads to sore, spongy gums; loose teeth; fragile blood vessels; swollen joints; and anemia. Signs also include interference with bone growth and slowed tissue repair.

Hormonal influences
Sex hormones

Sex hormones influence the time of the appearance of the ossification centers and stimulate closure of the epiphyses. These hormones initially stimulate bone growth during puberty, when their production is increased. This stimulation accounts for the growth spurts seen during this time of adolescence. However, the hormones also stimulate fusion

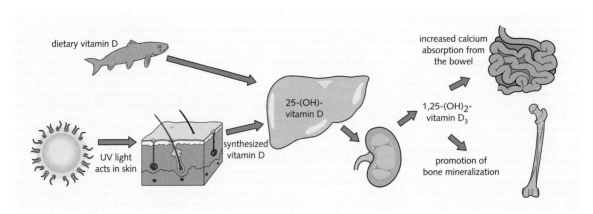

Fig. 4.13 Formation and actions of vitamin D.

of epiphyseal plates so that growth stops. Estrogens cause quicker ossification of the epiphyseal plates than does testosterone, which is why girls stop growing earlier than boys and are normally shorter than boys.

Precocious sexual development caused by hormone-secreting tumors or administration of sex hormones tends to retard growth by causing early epiphyseal closure; however, deficiencies of sex hormones caused by abnormal gonadal development tend to delay epiphyseal closure, prolonging the growth phase and resulting in tall stature.

Low estrogen levels, common in immobilized patients and postmenopausal women, give rise to osteoporosis. Although bone morphology is normal in patients with osteoporosis, patients experience a net decrease in bone mass caused by less bone formation and more bone resorption.

Growth hormone

Growth hormone is a peptide hormone released from the anterior pituitary gland to increase general tissue growth. The hormone is regulated by the growth hormone-releasing hormone and the inhibiting hormone, somatostatin. Growth hormone stimulates interstitial cartilage growth and appositional bone growth.

During the growing years, the release of too much growth hormone abnormally increases the length of long bone, resulting in gigantism. Adults with elevated growth hormone levels have acromegaly. In acromegaly, the epiphyseal plates have fused so that the bones cannot grow in length and instead become wider. A lack of growth hormone gives rise to pituitary dwarfism.

Thyroid hormones

Thyroid hormones regulate gene expression, metabolism, and the general development of all tissues. Triiodothyronine (T_3) and tetraiodothyronine (T_4) are peptide hormones released by the follicular cells of the thyroid gland. They are regulated by the thyroid-stimulating hormone (TSH) that is released from the anterior pituitary. Thyroid hormone deficiency in neonates leads to cretinism and associated dwarfism.

Hematopoiesis in bone

Hematopoiesis is the formation of mature blood cells from precursors. In humans, hematopoiesis occurs in the medullary cavities of bone. Red bone marrow is actively hematopoietic, while yellow bone marrow, (formerly red marrow), has become filled with adipocytes and is therefore inactive. When stress is applied to the hematopoietic system, yellow bone marrow can revert to red marrow.

Although the number of active sites of blood production in bone marrow lessens from birth to maturity, all bone marrow retains some hematopoietic potential. Hematopoietic activity can reappear in anemia and extramedullary hematopoiesis.

Location of hematopoiesis

In humans, hematopoiesis takes place in various sites according to the stage of development. In the embryo, primitive blood cells arise in the yolk sac within 4 weeks of conception.

At gestational week 6, the embryonic liver becomes the major site of hematopoiesis. The spleen and lymph nodes also show some activity. Bone marrow starts to produce blood cells when bones form medullary cavities after gestational week 20; bone is the only site to do so by birth, when all marrow is red.

In children, the diaphyses of long bone, but not the epiphyses, show replacement of red marrow by yellow marrow. In adults, hematopoiesis occurs only in some bones (e.g., the vertebrae, sternum, ribs, clavicles, proximal parts of the humerus, hip bones, and proximal parts of the femur) (Fig. 4.14).

The bone marrow receives its blood supply from vessels that supply cancellous bone. Nutrient arteries enter the midshaft of bone through the periosteum and pass through compact bone to reach the medullary space.

Response of bone to stress

Within limits, bone is a labile tissue that is capable of remodeling its internal structure according to different stresses (Fig. 4.15).

The two main mechanical stresses on bone are those from:
- The pull of skeletal muscles.
- The pull of gravity.

In response to mechanical stress, the increased deposition of mineral salts and production of collagen fibers make the bone stronger. In sites that are stressed frequently, bone is thicker and develops heavier prominences, and the trabeculae are rearranged (Fig. 4.16). Stress also increases the

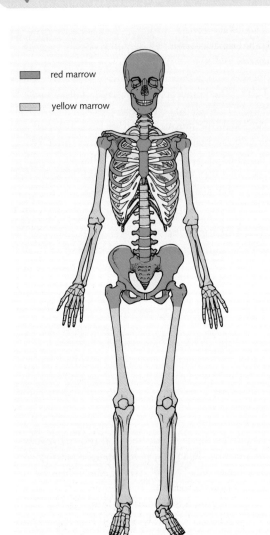

red marrow

yellow marrow

Fig. 4.14 Sites of hematopoiesis in an adult (adapted from *Anatomy and Physiology*, 3rd ed., by Seeley RR, Stephens TD, and Tate P, Mosby Year Book, 1995).

production of calcitonin, which inhibits bone resorption.

The bones of athletes, which are repeatedly subjected to high stresses, are notably thicker than those of nonathletes. Weight-bearing activities, such as walking, help build and retain bone mass. The removal of mechanical stress weakens bone through demineralization and collagen reduction. Bone is unable to remodel normally since resorption outstrips bone formation.

People who are bedridden or wear a cast lose strength in their unstressed bones. Astronauts subjected to the weightlessness of space also lose bone mass. In these situations, bone loss can be as much as 1% per week.

Disorders of bone

Hereditary abnormalities of bone
Osteogenesis imperfecta
Osteogenesis imperfecta, or brittle bone disease, is a group of disorders that may be inherited in several ways and have varying degrees of severity (Fig. 4.17). The genes responsible for osteogenesis imperfecta are found on chromosomes 7 and 17. The incidence of osteogenesis imperfecta is 1 in 20,000.

Pathology
In osteogenesis imperfecta, there is an abnormal synthesis of type I collagen that makes up 90% of bone matrix. Some forms of the disorder are fatal in the perinatal period; other forms predispose individuals to fractures, but there is a good survival rate overall.

Morphology
Osteopenia (decreased bone) occurs in osteogenesis imperfecta. This condition involves thinning of the cortex and trabeculae.

Other features
Other features of osteogenesis imperfecta include uveal pigment (blue) that can be seen through thin sclerae, deafness, and dental abnormalities. The prognosis is variable and depends on the severity of the disease.

Osteopetrosis
Osteopetrosis, also known as Albers-Schönberg or marble bone disease, is a group of rare inherited disorders of different severities (Fig. 4.18). If the condition is autosomal recessive, it presents from birth as anemia and leukocytopenia. Adult types predispose to fractures and infection.

Pathology
Osteopetrosis is a defect in osteoclast function that leads to decreased bone resorption and net bone overgrowth.

Morphology
In patients with osteopetrosis, there is overgrowth and sclerosis of bone, marked thickening of cortex,

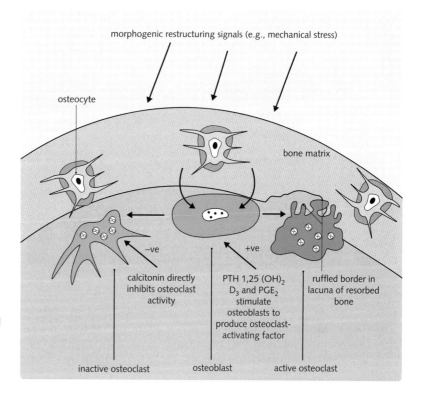

Fig. 4.15 Factors affecting bone remodeling in response to stress. (1,25[OH]$_2$D$_3$, 1,25-dihydroxyvitamin D$_3$; PGE$_2$, prostaglandin E$_2$; PTH, parathyroid hormone) (adapted from *Essential Endocrinology*, by Laycock J and Wise P, Oxford University Press, 1996).

morphogenic restructuring signals (e.g., mechanical stress)

osteocyte

bone matrix

−ve

+ve

calcitonin directly inhibits osteoclast activity

PTH 1,25 (OH)$_2$ D$_3$ and PGE$_2$ stimulate osteoblasts to produce osteoclast-activating factor

ruffled border in lacuna of resorbed bone

inactive osteoclast

osteoblast

active osteoclast

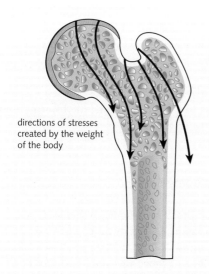

directions of stresses created by the weight of the body

Fig. 4.16 Orientation of trabeculae along lines of stress (adapted from *Anatomy and Physiology*, 3rd ed., by Seeley RR, Stephens TD, and Tate P, Mosby Year Book, 1995).

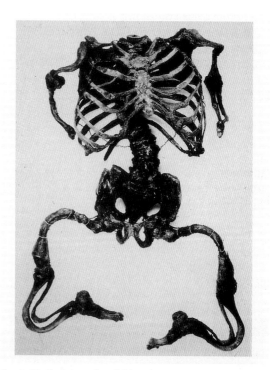

Fig. 4.17 Skeleton of a child with osteogenesis imperfecta congenita. Note the deformed limbs, scoliosis, and chest and pelvic deformities (courtesy of Dr. G Bullough and Dr. VJ Vigorita).

and narrowing and filling of the medullary cavity (inhibits hematopoiesis). Treatment involves bone marrow transplant. In the severe form, mental

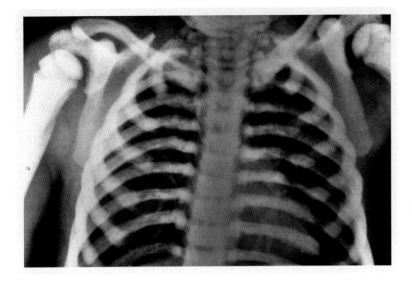

Fig. 4.18 Radiograph of the upper body of a child with osteopetrosis, showing a marked increase in density of all the bones (courtesy of Dr. G Bullough and Dr. VJ Vigorita).

retardation and early death may occur; in the mild form, changes in radiography may be the only detectable signs of the disease.

Achondroplasia

Achondroplasia is also known as dwarfism. It is a disorder caused by a single gene inherited in an autosomal dominant manner with complete penetrance. The incidence of achondroplasia is 1 in 25,000. Individuals who are homozygotes die soon after birth, whereas those who are heterozygotes have a normal lifespan and experience normal mental, sexual, and reproductive development.

Pathology

Patients with achondroplasia experience derangement of endochondral ossification.

Morphology

Those who are achondroplastic heterozygotes have short limbs and a normal-sized trunk. The person has an enlarged skull and has a big forehead and depression of the nasal bridge. The epiphyses are abnormally wide (appositional growth is unaffected).

Malformations

Occasionally, malformations of the bones in the skeleton occur in individuals with achondroplasia. These result from various factors:

- Failure of formation.
- Extra bones (in fingers and toes).
- Fusion of bones (skull sutures).

Generally, these malformations are of no consequence. However, correction is possible for cosmetic reasons.

Infections and trauma

Osteomyelitis

Osteomyelitis, or infection of bone, can be caused by any bacterial agent, especially in people who are immunosuppressed (Fig. 4.19).

Pyogenic osteomyelitis
Causes
In immunocompromised people, pyogenic osteomyelitis can be caused by *Staphylococcus aureus*, *Escherichia coli*, *Klebsiella* spp., *Pseudomonas* spp., *Salmonellae* spp., *Haemophilus influenzae*, and *Streptococcus* spp.

Spread
Spread of infection into bone can be by blood, local tissues, open fracture, or surgery. In developing countries, the spread of infection is usually hematogenous; in developed countries, it is usually due to trauma.

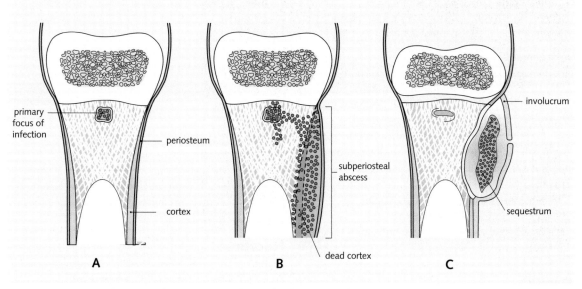

primary focus of infection

periosteum

cortex

subperiosteal abscess

dead cortex

involucrum

sequestrum

A   **B**   **C**

Fig. 4.19 Sequence of osteomyelitis. A. Primary focus of infection that has spread through bone, causing the death of cortical bone. B. Formation of a subperiosteal abscess. C. Death of a segment of bone (sequestrum), with the area being surrounded by new subperiosteal bone (involucrum).

Histology

Infection of bone leads to ischemic necrosis, fibrosis, and bony repair. The focus of infection starts initially around small vessels in the metaphysis. Necrosis of a bone segment is known as a sequestrum. This is surrounded by a sheath of subperiosteal new bone called the involucrum. Very sclerotic new bone forms a pattern called Garré's sclerosing osteomyelitis. There may be formation of sinus tracts or abscesses called Brodie's abscesses (these are sometimes sterile).

Clinical features

Infection of bone causes acute bone pain and fever. The infection usually starts in the metaphysis, where the rich blood supply encourages bacterial growth and enables spread to other areas. A lytic area surrounded by a zone of reactive new bone can be seen on radiographs.

Complications

Complications of bone infection include sinus tracts to the skin surface (called cloacae), fracture, septicemia, endocarditis, pyogenic arthritis, and an alteration in growth rate.

Management

Antibiotic treatment is critical to the management of pyogenic osteomyelitis. If a diagnosis is suspected, intravenous antibiotics against the most likely causative organisms should be started immediately.

Once the culture is identified from appropriate tissue or pus samples, the antibiotics can be adjusted accordingly. The course should include 2 weeks of intravenous antibiotics and 4 weeks of an oral dose. Surgery should be undertaken only if dead bone is present; dead bone can act as a nidus of infection and may lead to recurrence.

Tuberculous osteomyelitis

Tuberculous osteomyelitis is relatively uncommon in people who are immunocompetent. About 2% of all cases of tuberculosis have bone involvement.

Spread

Tuberculous osteomyelitis is spread hematogenously. It is more destructive and resistant to control than the pyogenic form.

Clinical features

Tuberculous osteomyelitis is usually a chronic condition with involvement of a single bone (except in patients with AIDS). It usually occurs in long bones and in the thoracic and lumbar vertebrae, where it is called Pott's disease.

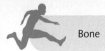

Complications

Tuberculous osteomyelitis causes fractures, nerve compression, and tuberculous arthritis.

Management

The management of tuberculous osteomyelitis is both medical and surgical. Combination chemotherapy with rifampicin, isoniazid, and para-aminosalicylic acid is administered during the course of several months under the guidance of infectious disease specialists. Debridement of infected bones and joints reduces the amount of infectious material present.

If the spine is involved, prolonged bed rest, administration of a plaster cast to prevent deformity, and surgical stabilization may be required.

Syphilis

Syphilis in the skeleton

Syphilis of bone can be either congenital or acquired (Fig. 4.20). The condition is rare because of its early treatment with penicillin.

Histology

In syphilis of bone, local periostitis leads to new bone formation on the outer cortex. Gummata are the characteristic lesions of syphilis. They have a center of rubbery, gray-white coagulation necrosis surrounded by epithelioid or fibroblastic cells.

Clinical features

On radiographs of affected skulls, the effects of syphilis are seen as a "crew-cut" outline. When the tibia is involved, there is a "saber shin" appearance. The destruction and collapse of nasal and parietal bones can create a "saddle nose."

Treatment

Syphilis is treated with penicillin, usually for 2 weeks, but treatment may be extended to 3 weeks when the disease presents in the late stage. For patients allergic to penicillin, tetracycline or erythromycin is also effective.

Fractures

Types

There are several types of bone fractures:
- Simple (clean break).
- Comminuted (multiple bone fragments).
- Compound (breaks through overlying skin).
- Stress (small linear fragments).
- Pathologic (bones weakened by disease).
- Greenstick (partial break).

Causes

Fractures are usually caused by trauma, which is either substantial or minor and repeated. Pathologic fractures arise from disease (e.g., tumors, osteoporosis, Paget's disease, osteomalacia).

Healing

Healing of fractures requires immobilization of approximated bone ends and good alignment.

Delayed or imperfect healing

The delayed or imperfect healing of bone fractures can be caused by malalignment, movement during healing, poor blood supply, and soft tissue interposition in the fracture gap. These conditions can occur in the elderly, those in poor general health, and people who are immunosuppressed.

Histology of healing

Healing of a fracture follows a sequence (Fig. 4.21). The histologic changes that take place during healing include:
- Development of a hematoma, which forms a soft procallus (Fig. 4.21, A).
- Conversion of the procallus to a fibrocartilaginous callus (Fig. 4.21, B).

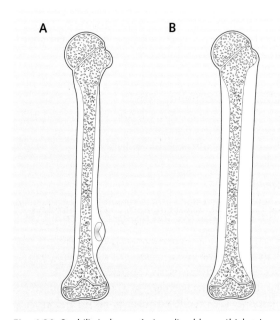

Fig. 4.20 Syphilis in bone. A. Localized bone thickening. B. Diffuse bone thickening.

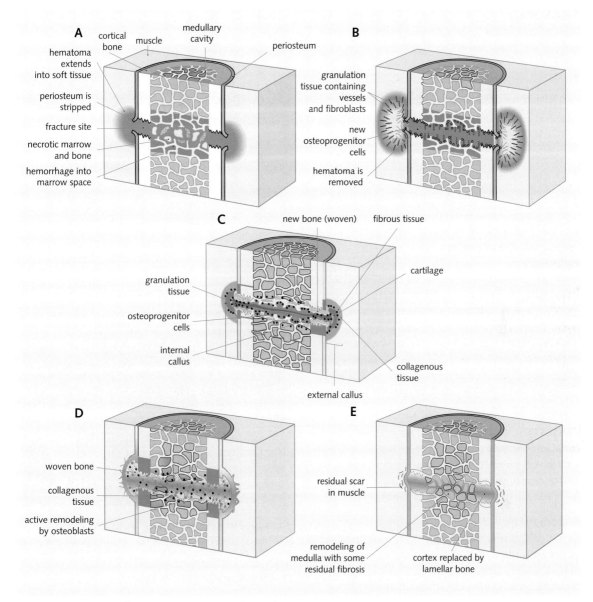

Fig. 4.21 Sequence of fracture repair. See text for explanation.

- Replacement of a fibrocartilaginous callus to an osseous callus—trabecular lamellar bone (Figs 4.21, C and D).
- Remodeling along weight-bearing lines by osteoclasts (Fig. 4.21, E).

Complications

Complications of fractures can include malunion of bones, avascular necrosis, shock, osteoarthritis, infection, and deep vein thrombosis.

Management

The immediate management of fractures involves immobilization of the fracture, coverage of the wound with a sterile dressing, and pain relief. Individual management of fractures depends on the age and expectation of the patient, the pathology present, and the patient's personal requirements in terms of occupation and other such factors. The basic principles of fracture management are as follows:

- Reduction of the deformity, replacing the bone fragments in their previous anatomic position— external or internal fixation may be necessary to achieve this goal.
- Maintenance of the reduction until the fractured bone reunites either by a plaster cast, brace, and/ or traction.
- Encouraging the healing of the fracture and surrounding structures by providing optimum conditions.
- Rehabilitation, including early mobilization of adjacent joints to prevent stiffness and wasting.
- Minimization of complications (see previous paragraphs).

Avascular necrosis
Pathology
Avascular necrosis involves the death of bone and marrow without infection and is caused by a poor blood supply. It is mostly seen in the head of the femur (intrascapular fractures) and scaphoid, occurring when fractures deprive adjacent areas of their blood supply (Fig. 4.22). Medullary infarctions affect cancellous bone and bone marrow, with cortical sparing. Subchondral infarctions lead to wedge-shaped areas of damage.

Causes
Avascular necrosis can be idiopathic or caused by trauma, thromboembolism, sickle-cell disease, polycythemia, immunosuppression, or decompression sickness (seen in scuba divers).

Histology
Dead bone is identified by empty lacunae surrounded by necrotic adipocytes. The adipocytes may rupture to release fatty acids that will bind calcium and form deposits. Osteoclastic resorption of trabeculae occurs, and the articular cartilage is distorted.

Clinical features
Pain and immobility are present in avascular necrosis. The patient cannot walk, especially if the condition is a complication of fracture (most commonly seen in older adults).

Metabolic diseases of bone

Osteoporosis
Osteoporosis is a very common disease of older adults, especially postmenopausal women, resulting in abnormally decreased bone mass.

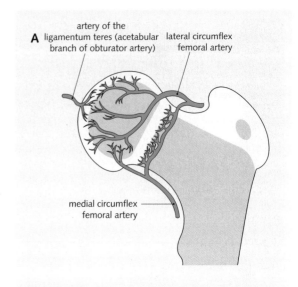

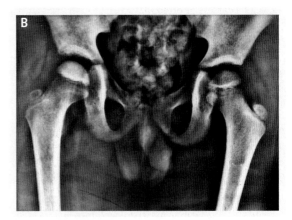

Fig. 4.22 Avascular necrosis of the femoral head (Perthe's disease). A. Normal blood supply. B. Radiograph showing widened joint space, cessation of growth of the bony epiphyses, and increased growth of cartilage (courtesy of Dr. PG Bullough and Dr. VJ Vigorita).

Classification
Osteoporosis can be localized or generalized and can be classified as primary or secondary:
- Primary osteoporosis occurs in old age and postmenopausal women.
- Secondary osteoporosis is caused by endocrine abnormalities, gut malabsorption, and neoplasia.

Histology
In an individual with osteoporosis, the bone cortex has thinned, the trabeculae are attenuated, and there are wide haversian canals (Fig. 4.23). Increased osteoclastic resorption with slowed bone formation

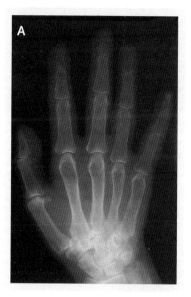
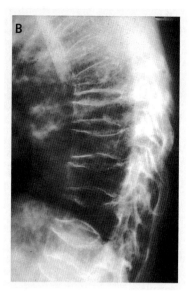
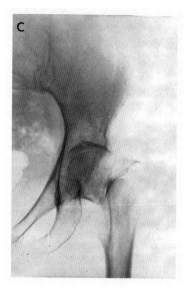

Fig. 4.23 Features of osteoporosis. A. Loss of cortical thickening and reduction of trabeculae in the hand. B. Wedge-shaped flattening of vertebral bodies leading to loss of height. C. Fracture of the neck of the femur in an older adult (courtesy of Dr. PG Bullough and Dr. VJ Vigorita).

occurs. The main sites affected are the vertebrae, femoral necks, wrists, and pelvis. In the spine, there may be disc herniation and nerve root compression.

Etiology
Possible causes of osteoporosis include decreased exercise or immobilization; estrogen deficiency; lack of calcium, vitamin D, or fluoride; hyperadrenocorticism; hypogonadism; thyrotoxicosis; hypopituitarism; pregnancy; diabetes; and long-term heparin administration.

Clinical features
Osteoporosis causes bone pain, loss of height, fractures, and deformities such as exaggerated cervical and lumbar lordosis and dorsal kyphosis. Diagnosis is achieved by bone density scans or a biopsy. A 30% loss of bone mass is required before radiographs show translucency.

Clinical consequences include:
- Pain.
- Increased mortality (especially in the first year following hip fractures).
- Vertebral crush fractures.
- Deformity (loss of height, kyphosis, lordosis).
- Loss of independence.

Treatment for osteoporosis includes hormone replacement to increase estrogen levels and exercise to strengthen weight-bearing joints.

Management
The rapid bone loss in postmenopausal women may be countered to some extent by hormone replacement therapy (HRT); HRT should be maintained for a minimum of 5 years to be useful in preventing osteoporosis. Bisphosphonates inhibit osteoclast action and increase bone density. They may be given orally or intravenously. Protracted treatment with calcium and vitamin D has also been proven to reduce the risk of fracture.

Rickets and osteomalacia
Rickets occurs in growing children, and osteomalacia develops in adults. These conditions are caused by either a vitamin D deficiency or phosphate depletion—the latter cause is less common.

Etiology
Vitamin D deficiency can be caused by low quantities in the diet, insufficient exposure to sunlight, malabsorption, or deranged liver or kidney metabolism. Phosphate depletion can be caused by X-linked phosphatemia, neoplasia, or poisoning from heavy metals.

Pathology
Rickets and osteomalacia arise from a failure of bone mineralization, which leads to softer and wider

channels of matrix. Excess unmineralized matrix and underdeveloped epiphyseal cartilage calcification lead to endochondral bone that is deranged and overgrown.

Clinical features

Rickets presents with bowing of the legs, overgrowth of costochondral junctions (forming a "rachitic rosary"), widened epiphyses, and either a flattened ("bossed") square skull or craniotabes (the skull snaps back into shape after being pressed in) (Fig. 4.24).

Osteomalacia presents with spontaneous incomplete fractures ("Looser's zones") in long bones and the pelvis, bone pain, weakened proximal limb muscles, and a decreased level of serum calcium. Bone biopsy is needed to confirm the diagnosis of rickets or osteomalacia. Treatment involves oral or intravenous administration of vitamin D and an improved diet.

Management

Treatment involving vitamin D (with adequate phosphate intake) and calcium regulates bone formation and is used in the management of rickets and osteomalacia. Corrective osteotomies may also be required if the deformities are severe and established.

Hypercalcemia, which leads to muscle weakness, lethargy, confusion, polyuria, and dehydration, is caused by hyperparathyroidism or bone malignancy caused by metastatic bone disease or multiple myeloma. Less common causes include thyrotoxicosis, sarcoidosis, and an excess level of vitamin D. It is important to be aware of this condition because severe hypercalcemia leads to crisis, the main features of which are gross dehydration resulting from polyuria. It is treated by rehydration and intravenous bisphosphonate to reduce the loss of bone calcium.

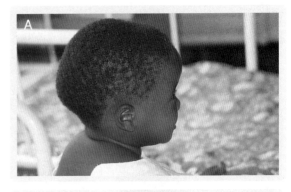

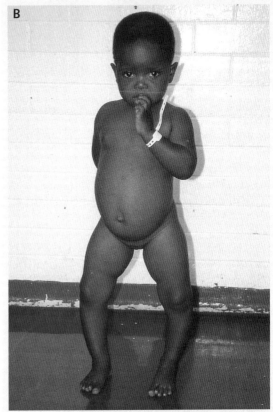

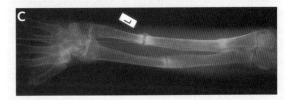

Fig. 4.24 Rickets and osteomalacia. A. Skull "bossing" in rickets patient. B. Lateral and forward bowing of legs in rickets patient. C. Radiograph showing pseudofractures (Looser's zones) in the forearm in osteomalacia (A and B courtesy of Dr. S. Taylor and Dr. A. Raffles; C courtesy of Dr. PG Bullough and Dr VJ Vigorita).

Hyperparathyroidism

Classification

Hyperparathyroidism can be:

- Primary—caused by a lesion of the parathyroid gland, which increases PTH and thus raises calcium levels.
- Secondary—owing to bone metastases, inappropriate PTH secretion by tumors, or renal failure (normal or lowered serum calcium).
- Tertiary—caused by the development of an autonomous adenoma in the parathyroid glands, which occurs following the persistent hyperactivity of the glands as they secrete PTH.

Pathology

Increased PTH levels cause an increase in osteoclast activity, leading to increased bone resorption.

Histology

In hyperparathyroidism, demineralization leads to increased osteoclast activity and resorption. The patient experiences characteristic peritrabecular fibrosis, called osteitis fibrosa, and more marked fibrosis and cyst formation within the marrow (osteitis fibrosa cystica or von Recklinghausen's disease of the bone). "Brown tumors" of osteoclasts, fibrosis, and hemorrhage are also seen (Fig. 4.25). These resemble giant-cell granulomas.

Clinical features

In hyperparathyroidism, radiographs of the phalanges and clavicles show "moth-eaten" erosions (see Fig. 4.25). This bone damage can be reversed by treating the cause of the excess PTH.

Management

Primary and tertiary hyperparathyroidism conditions are treated by parathyroidectomy after the affected gland has been identified by biopsy. In secondary hyperparathyroidism, a subtotal parathyroidectomy is performed, which involves removal of three-and-a-half of the four glands. Surgical risks include inducing hypocalcemia if too much gland tissue is removed and damage to the recurrent laryngeal nerve.

Renal osteodystrophy

Renal osteodystrophy is the collective term for all the skeletal changes occurring in a patient with chronic renal disease.

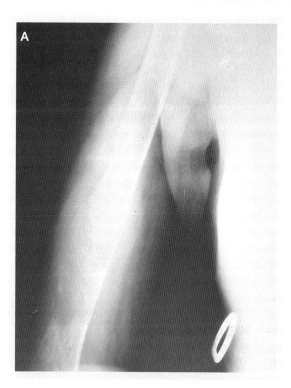

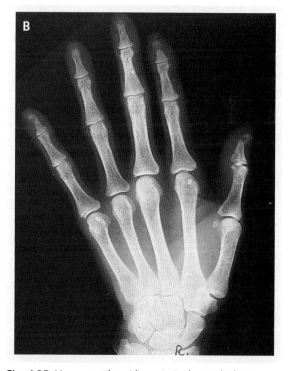

Fig. 4.25 Hyperparathyroidism. A. Radiograph showing large destructive lesion ("brown tumor") in the lower half of the humerus (courtesy of Dr. PG Bullough).
B. Radiograph showing subperiosteal erosion of the cortical surfaces of the phalanges (courtesy of Dr. A Norman).

Pathology

Renal osteodystrophy is caused by:

- Inadequate renal tissue for making vitamin D—leads to osteomalacia.
- High serum phosphate—precipitates hyperparathyroidism.
- Prolonged hemodialysis—inhibits calcification of bone matrix and produces osteomalacia.
- Steroids—may induce osteoporosis or avascular necrosis.

Clinical features

The clinical features and management of renal osteodystrophy are similar to those of osteitis fibrosa cystica and osteomalacia. Osteosclerosis occurs, and chronically there are metastatic calcifications in the skin, eyes, joints, and arterial walls.

Tumors of the skeleton

Metastatic tumors of the skeleton

Metastatic tumors of the skeleton are much more common than primary bone tumors, particularly in adults. Metastases arising from the breast, lung, kidney, and thyroid are lytic, whereas those from the prostate are sclerotic.

Cartilage-forming tumors
Chondroma and endochondroma

Cartilage-forming tumors are benign tumors composed of mature hyaline cartilage. Those within bone are endochondromas, and those on the surface are subperiosteal chondromas (Fig. 4.26).

Epidemiology

Males are more likely than females to develop cartilage-forming tumors; these tumors usually develop between 20 and 50 years of age.

Classification

There are two types of cartilage-forming tumors: solitary and multiple. Multiple tumors involve nonfamilial types (enchondromatosis or Ollier's disease) and familial types (Maffucci's syndrome). Familial types are associated with hemangiomas.

Clinical features

Features of cartilage-forming tumors include bone pain and fractures. The tumors consist of cartilage nests and arise at the epiphyses. There is a risk of chondrosarcoma in multiple lesions, especially if the condition is familial.

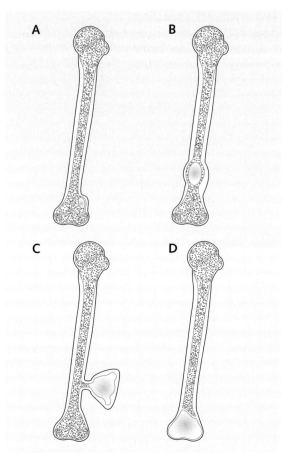

Fig. 4.26 Benign bone tumors. A. Osteoma. B. Endochondroma and chondroma. C. Osteochondroma. D. Giant-cell tumor.

Management

Many of these lesions do not require treatment. When needed, treatment consists of curettage of the cartilage tissue and the grafting of bone onto the subsequent defect.

Chondrosarcoma

Chondrosarcomas are malignant tumors of cartilage. They grow slowly and occur half as frequently as osteosarcomas—75% are primary, and the rest form endochondromas, osteochondromas, and chondroblastomas.

Epidemiology

Males are more likely than females to develop chondrosarcomas, and these tumors usually develop when the individual is more than 30 years of age.

Classification
Chondrosarcomas are graded from 1 to 3 according to nuclear atypia. Five-year survival rates range from 90% (low grade) to 40% (high grade).

Clinical features
Radiographs of chondrosarcomas show localized areas of bone destruction mottled with dense calcified spots. High-grade tumors spread hematogenously, notably to the lungs. Typical sites are central bones, such as the pelvis, scapula, and ribs. Histology shows large, gelatinous, lobulated tumors that are translucent when cut; necrosis; and spotty calcifications.

Chondroblastoma
Chondroblastomas, or Codman's tumors, are rare benign tumors that affect the epiphyses of young people. The tumors, which are composed of chondroblasts arranged in sheets, have a grooved nucleus and a surrounding calcified network; osteoclast-like cells may also be present.

Chondromyxoid fibroma
Chondromyxoid fibromas are rare benign tumors composed of cartilage matrix and fibrous and myxoid tissue.

Epidemiology
Males are more likely than females to develop chondromyxoid fibromas, and they usually occur between 10 and 30 years of age.

Clinical features
Radiographs of chondromyxoid fibromas show circumscribed lucencies with scattered calcifications, usually in the metaphyses of the tibia, fibula, and humerus.

Bone-forming tumors
Osteochondroma
Osteochondromas, or exostoses, are benign mushroom-shaped outgrowths of bone capped with cartilage and attached to the skeleton by a bony stalk. Osteochondromas can grow up to 20 cm in diameter.

Epidemiology
Males are more likely than females to develop osteochondromas than females; development of the outgrowths usually occurs when the individual is less than 20 years of age.

Classification
There are two types of osteochondroma:
- Solitary, developing in young adults.
- Multiple, developing in children and inherited in an autosomal-dominant pattern.

Clinical features
In osteochondroma, lesions are near the epiphyses of long bones. Malignant change is rare but can occur in multiple lesions.

Management
Simple excision is the definitive treatment for osteochondromas.

Osteoma
Osteomas are slow-growing benign tumors composed of sclerotic bone that is well formed (see Fig. 4.26). Osteomas are unlikely to become malignant.

Epidemiology
Both young and middle-aged people can develop osteomas.

Classification
There are two types of osteoma:
- Solitary, developing in middle age.
- Multiple, developing in young people and often associated with polyposis coli (Gardner's syndrome).

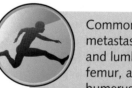
Common sites of bony metastases include the thoracic and lumbar spine, the proximal femur, and the proximal humerus. Patients often present with pathologic fractures—breaks in the bone caused by minimal stress. Patients may also present with hypercalcemia.

Clinical features
Osteomas are likely to protrude from cortical surfaces, especially the skull and facial bones. They are usually harmless unless the location compromises organ function (e.g., intracranial growth in the skull).

Osteoid osteoma and osteoblastoma
Osteoid osteomas are small benign tumors surrounded by a dense sclerotic ring of new bone and

are usually less than 2 cm in diameter.
Osteoblastomas (also called giant osteoid osteomas)
have a similar histology, without the sclerotic ring,
and are usually more than 2 cm in diameter.

Epidemiology
Males are more likely than females to develop
osteoid osteomas and osteoblastomas; these usually
develop between 5 and 25 years of age.

Clinical features
Osteoid osteomas are located in the cortex of the tibia
and femur and are very painful. Radiographs show a
small radiolucent "nest" of trabecular bone
surrounded by a ring of dense sclerotic bone. The nest
consists of osteoid, osteoblasts, and a vascular stroma.

Osteoblastomas are less painful than osteoid
osteomas and are found in the vertebrae and long
bones. They may become malignant and form
osteosarcomas.

In all patients with back pain,
especially pain that is
unremitting and frequently
severe at night, the most likely
primary tumor sites—lung and
breast—must be assessed. In men over
the age of 45, the prostate must also
be assessed.

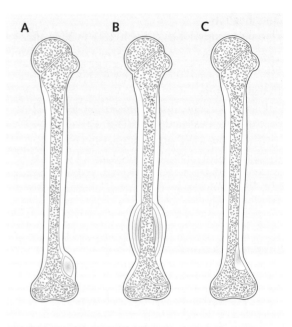

Fig. 4.27 Malignant bone tumors. A. Osteosarcoma.
B. Ewing's sarcoma. C. Metastatic bone tumors.

Osteosarcoma
Osteosarcomas are the most common type of
primary bone tumor (Fig. 4.27). They are composed
of osteocytes and osteoid. Osteosarcomas are
thought to be related to the retinoblastoma and p53
genes. They grow quickly and, with combination
therapy, have a 60% 5-year survival rate. Some
histological variants, such as juxtacortical and
periosteal types, have a better prognosis.

Epidemiology
Males are more likely than females to develop
osteosarcomas; these can occur up to 20 years of age,
although older adults with pre-existing bone tumors
are also at risk.

Clinical features
Osteosarcomas are found in the medullary cavity of
metaphyses of long bones (especially near the knee);
they are also found in flat bones of older adults.
Osteosarcomas produce bone pain, tenderness, and
swelling and are usually a complication of Paget's
disease of bone. Radiographs show elevated
periosteum (Codman's triangle) caused by new bone
growth under the periosteum. There may be
hematogenous spread to the lungs.

Management
During the past 25 years, new multidrug
chemotherapy has been introduced, which has
led to a reduction in the mortality rate of
patients with osteosarcomas. The adoption of
aggressive surgical treatment has also led to an
increase in patient survival; cure rates vary but
may reach up to 80%.

Fibrous and fibro-osseous tumors
Fibroma
Fibromas are benign, well-defined tumors
composed of fibroblasts and collagenous tissue. They
are usually found in the ovary but may develop
elsewhere.

Fibrous dysplasia
Fibrous dysplasia is a benign disorder in which there
is progressive replacement of bone. This takes place
by fibroblasts that are arranged in a regular pattern
with small spicules of immature bone. As a result, the
bones become structurally weakened.

Epidemiology
Fibrous dysplasia affects children and young adults.

Classification
There are three types of fibrous dysplasia:
- Monostotic (70%).
- Polyostotic (25%).
- Polyostotic associated with endocrinopathies (5%).

Albright's syndrome is fibrous dysplasia with precocious sexual development and irregular skin pigmentation.

Clinical features
Fibrous dysplasia is found in the ribs, femur, tibia, and skull. There is a "ground glass" appearance on radiographs and *café-au-lait* spots over affected bones. Rarely, some can become osteosarcomas.

Miscellaneous tumors
Ewing's sarcoma
Ewing's sarcomas are aggressive malignant round cell tumors of uncertain histogenesis, although it is thought to be of neuroectodermal orgin (see Fig. 4.27). These tumors contain small, round or ovoid cells growing in sheets around blood vessels and show focal necrosis and hemorrhage. However, they respond to drugs (multimodal chemotherapy) and have an overall 5-year survival of 60%. The tumor metastasizes to lungs and lymph nodes.

Epidemiology
Females are more likely than males to develop Ewing's sarcoma usually when they are less than 25 years of age. Ewing's sarcoma is very rare in Afro-Caribbean children.

Clinical features
Ewing's sarcoma presents as a soft-tissue mass—periosteal "onion-skinning" is seen on radiographs. This is often followed by a "moth-eaten" or mottled appearance of the bone and is accompanied by the extension of the lesion into soft tissue.

Management
Treatment for Ewing's sarcoma is medical and surgical. Preoperatively, multimodal chemotherapy with vincristine, dactinomycin, and cyclophosphamide (VAC) and radiation are used. Following tumor resection, chemotherapy is used to reduce the chance of recurrence.

Giant-cell tumor
Giant-cell tumors, or osteoclastomas, are low-grade malignant tumors of giant multinucleate cells and stroma; about 10% form metastases (see Fig. 4.26).

Epidemiology
Females are more likely than males to develop giant-cell tumors; these develop usually between 20 and 40 years of age.

Clinical features
Radiographs of giant-cell tumors show large lytic "soap-bubble" lesions with absent calcified spots. These can often be mistaken for "brown tumors" that occur in patients with hyperparathyroidism. Giant-cell tumors are found at the metaphyses and epiphyses of long bones, especially the knees.

Management
The treatment and management of giant-cell tumors depend on the history and histologic grading of the lesion. Recommended methods of removal include curettage and bone grafting as well as cryosurgery involving the use of liquid nitrogen to destroy residual tumor cells.

Treatment of bone pain caused by tumors is palliative. Bones that are at risk for fracture because of malignant pathology are often treated prophylactically by internal fixation because the risk of fracture is substantial if more than one third of the bone's width is destroyed by tumor lesions.

Other diseases of bone

Paget's disease of bone
Paget's disease of bone is also known as osteitis deformans. It is a disease of disordered bone formation and resorption. It commonly occurs in people who are more than 40 years of age and affects males more than females. Paget's disease of bone usually occurs in white populations of the Western world; it is rare in Asians and Africans.

Classification
Paget's disease of bone affects either one bone (15%) or several (85%). Bones usually affected are the tibia, femur, ileum, vertebrae, humerus, and skull (Fig. 4.28).

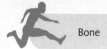

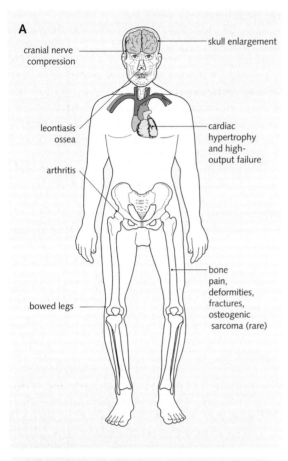

cranial nerve compression

skull enlargement

leontiasis ossea

cardiac hypertrophy and high-output failure

arthritis

bowed legs

bone pain, deformities, fractures, osteogenic sarcoma (rare)

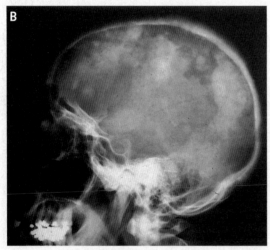

Fig. 4.28 Paget's disease of bone. A. General features. B. Radiograph of skull in late stage showing patchy sclerosis and loss of diploic architecture (courtesy of Dr. PG Bullough).

Causes

The cause of Paget's disease of bone is unknown, but the disease may develop from infection of osteoclasts by the paramyxovirus, measles virus, or respiratory syncytial virus.

Pathology

Paget's disease of bone occurs in three phases:
- Initial osteolytic phase, when there is a huge increase in osteoclastic activity.
- Mixed osteoclast/osteoblast phase, when there is disordered activity, and a mosaic pattern of bone is produced.
- Quiescent osteosclerotic phase, when new sclerotic bone is produced after a period of years.

Histology

In a patient with Paget's disease of bone, the bone is thickened but weak. Intertrabecular fibrosis and a mosaic pattern of new bone occur, and the osteoid is very bulky and porous.

Clinical features

Fractures and coarsened facial bones in patients with Paget's disease of bone lead to a leonine facies, bone pain, and fractures. A person may experience deafness because of nerve compression by the overgrown skull. Serum alkaline phosphatase and calcium levels are raised, and hydroxyproline is present in the urine.

Complications

Complications of Paget's disease of bone include secondary osteoarthritis, high-output heart failure caused by new blood vessels forming shunts, and Paget's sarcoma.

Management

Management is both medical and surgical. Salicylates and nonsteroidal anti-inflammatory drugs may reduce the plan. Etidronate disodium, synthetic salmon calcitonin, and biphosphates are used to inhibit osteoclast action and slow down the pathologic remodeling of bone. Surgical correction of severe deformities is also sometimes performed; because bone heals poorly in this condition, intramedullary fixation devices are usually applied at the end of the operation.

Hypertrophic pulmonary osteoarthropathy

Hypertrophic pulmonary osteoarthropathy is an uncommon, idiopathic condition causing changes to bones and joints.

Pathology

A patient with hypertrophic pulmonary osteoarthropathy experiences:

- New periosteal bone formation in the distal long bones, wrists, ankles, and proximal phalanges.
- Arthritis of adjacent joints.
- Clubbing of digits.

Clinical features

Hypertrophic pulmonary osteoarthropathy is associated with congenital heart disease, chronic pulmonary disease, lung cancer, or pleural mesothelioma. Almost 90% of cases are associated with lung cancer, and there is usually an increased blood flow to the bones.

Management

Resection of the tumors usually leads to regression of the condition.

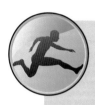

- List the functions of the skeleton.
- Describe the microstructure of the cartilage.
- Give a simple classification of cartilage type.
- Describe the microstructure of bone.
- Name two types of ossification.
- List the factors that affect bone growth.
- Describe remodeling of immature bone.
- Explain how calcium levels are maintained by PTH and calcium.
- List hormonal influences on bone.
- List the causes of hereditary abnormalities of bone.
- Describe the features of pyogenic osteomyelitis.
- List the different types of fracture and how they heal.
- Explain the causes and pathology of osteoporosis.
- Describe the difference between osteoporosis and osteomalacia.
- Give a simple classification of hyperparathyroidism and its effects.
- Describe the effects of renal disease on bone.
- Describe the features of Paget's disease of bone.
- Give a simple classification of tumors of the skeleton.
- Distinguish between benign and malignant tumors of bone.

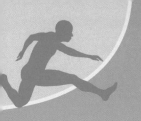

5. Joints and Related Structures

Classification of joints

Joints are the site at which two or more bones are united, regardless of whether there is movement between them. Joints are classified as fibrous, cartilaginous, or synovial according to the type of tissue between the bones (Figs. 5.1–5.3).

Fibrous

Fibrous joints have fibrous tissue uniting the bones. This type of joint allows very little movement.

Cartilaginous

There are two types of cartilaginous joints—primary and secondary.

Primary cartilaginous

Primary cartilaginous joints unite two bones with a plate of hyaline cartilage. No movement is possible with this type of joint.

Secondary cartilaginous

Secondary cartilaginous joints unite two bones with a plate of fibrocartilage; there is also a thin layer of

hyaline cartilage on the articular surfaces. A small amount of movement is possible with this type of joint.

Synovial

Synovial joints have a thin layer of hyaline cartilage on the articulating surfaces of the bones that are separated by a joint cavity and covered by a fibrous joint capsule. The cells of the synovial membrane lining the capsule secrete a lubricating nutritive medium called synovial fluid. An extensive range of movement is possible with this type of joint.

There are several types of synovial joints, and the different types are distinguished by the shape of the articulating surfaces and the range of movements possible.

Structure and function of joints

The structure and function of joints are closely related. The range of movements available at a joint is related to its stability. The stability depends on the shape, size, and arrangement of the bones; the strength and flexibility of the ligaments; and the tone of muscles around the joint.

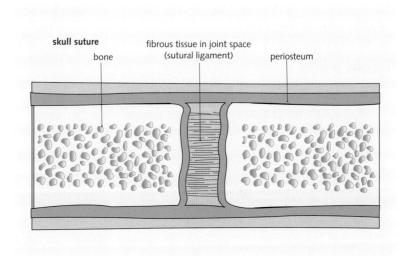

skull suture   fibrous tissue in joint space
bone   (sutural ligament)   periosteum

Fig. 5.1 Fibrous joint.

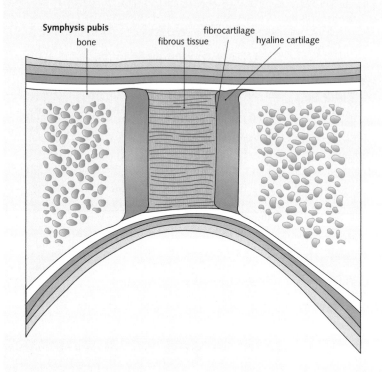

Fig. 5.2 Secondary cartilaginous joint.

Generally, the more stable a joint, the less movement it permits. If a joint is solid (no cavity), then it has limited mobility. If a cavity exists between the two ends of bone, movement can occur. Fibrous and cartilaginous joints are both known as synarthroses (i.e., solid joints). Synovial joints are diarthroses (i.e., cavitated joints).

Fibrous joints

Fibrous joints consist of two bones united by fibrous tissue. These types of joints have no cavity, and little or no movement is possible. Fibrous joints are further classified as sutures, syndesmoses, and gomphoses.

Sutures

Sutures are interdigitating bones held together by dense fibrous connective tissue. This type of joint occurs in the skull. The inner and outer layers of periosteum of the adjacent bones are continuous over the joint and through the joint space; these two layers and the fibrous tissue form the sutural ligament.

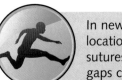

In newborns, at certain locations in the skull where the sutures meet, there are wide gaps covered with membrane; these are called "fontanelles." The flat bones of the skull vault (calvaria) undergo intramembranous ossification, forming a synostosis. This process occurs in normal adults between the frontal and parietal bones. However, beginning in a person's late twenties, fusion between the coronal, sagittal, and lambdoid sutures also begins.

Syndesmoses

Syndesmoses are where bones are separated by a larger distance than in sutures and are joined by a sheet of fibrous tissue—either a ligament or a membrane. This type of joint occurs in the radioulnar interosseous membrane.

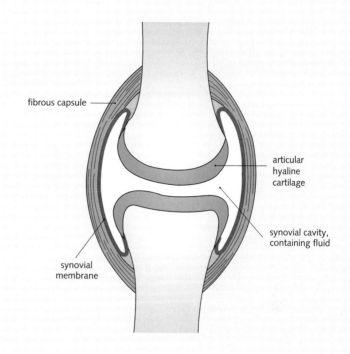

Fig. 5.3 Synovial joint.

A small amount of movement may be achieved with syndesmoses. The degree of movement depends on the distance between the bones and the flexibility of the fibrous ligaments.

Gomphoses

Gomphoses are specialized joints that occur between teeth and their sockets and the alveolar processes of the maxillae and mandible. Gomphoses are anchored by the fibrous tissue of the periodontal ligament. Movement of a gomphosis usually suggests a pathologic condition (e.g., disease loosening a tooth).

Primary cartilaginous joints

Primary cartilaginous joints are also known as synchondroses. The bones are united by hyaline cartilage. They are found in the epiphyseal growth plates and costochondral joints. Synchondroses appear in the normal development of long bones, so most are temporary unions. This type of joint is slightly moveable.

Secondary cartilaginous joints

Secondary cartilaginous joints are also known as symphyses. The articulating surfaces of the bone are covered with a thin layer of hyaline cartilage and joined by fibrocartilage. They are found in the manubriosternal joint, symphysis pubis, intervertebral discs, and the mandibular symphysis in the newborn. This type of joint is slightly moveable and is built for strength.

Synovial joints

Synovial joints are the most common joints in the skeleton and also the most functionally important of joints (Fig. 5.4). These joints are built essentially for mobility.

Fully formed synovial joints can be characterized by six features:
- The articular surfaces of the bones involved are covered by a thin layer of hyaline cartilage.
- A viscous synovial fluid provides lubrication.
- There is a joint cavity.
- The cavity is lined by synovial membrane.
- The joint is surrounded by a fibrous joint capsule.
- The capsule is reinforced externally or internally (or both) by fibrous ligaments.

Synovial joints are classified according to the shape of the articular surfaces of the bones involved and the

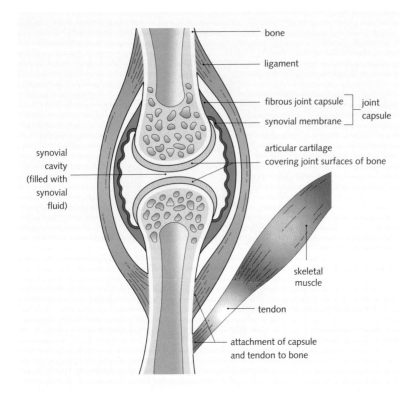

bone

ligament

fibrous joint capsule ⎤ joint
synovial membrane ⎦ capsule

articular cartilage
covering joint surfaces of bone

synovial
cavity
(filled with
synovial
fluid)

skeletal
muscle

tendon

attachment of capsule
and tendon to bone

Fig. 5.4 Features of a synovial joint. The articular cartilages and fluid-filled synovial cavity prevent bone from rubbing against bone.

movements that are possible. The movements at synovial joints can be described as:

- Monoaxial (i.e., occur in one direction or plane).
- Biaxial (i.e., occur in two directions or planes).
- Multiaxial (i.e., occur in many directions or planes).

Plane joints

Plane joints are shaped like two flat surfaces (Fig. 5.5, A). They allow a sliding movement (i.e., monoaxial). Examples of plane joints are the sternoclavicular and acromioclavicular joints.

Hinge joints

Hinge joints have concave and convex-shaped surfaces (Fig. 5.5, B). They allow flexion and extension movements (i.e., monoaxial). Examples of hinge joints are the elbow, knee, and ankle joints.

Pivot joints

Pivot joints consist of a cylindrical projection inside a ring (Fig. 5.5, C). They allow rotation movements (i.e., monoaxial). Examples of pivot joints are the atlantoaxial and proximal radioulnar joints.

Saddle joints

Saddle joints have concave and convex surfaces that are saddle-shaped (Fig. 5.5, D). They allow flexion, extension, abduction, and rotation movements (i.e., biaxial). The carpometacarpal (CMC) joint of the thumb is a saddle joint.

Ball-and-socket joints

Ball-and-socket joints are shaped like a ball sitting in a cup or a socket (Fig. 5.5, E). They allow flexion, extension, abduction, and medial and lateral rotation movements (i.e., multiaxial). Examples of ball-and-socket joints are the shoulder and the hip joints.

Ellipsoid joints

Ellipsoid joints have ellipsoid concave and convex surfaces (Fig. 5.5, F). They allow flexion, extension, abduction, and adduction movements but no rotation (i.e., biaxial). The wrist joint is an example of an ellipsoid joint.

Condyloid joints

Condyloid joints are shaped like two sets of concave and convex surfaces at right angles to each other (Fig. 5.5, G). They allow flexion, extension, abduction, adduction, and a small amount of rotation

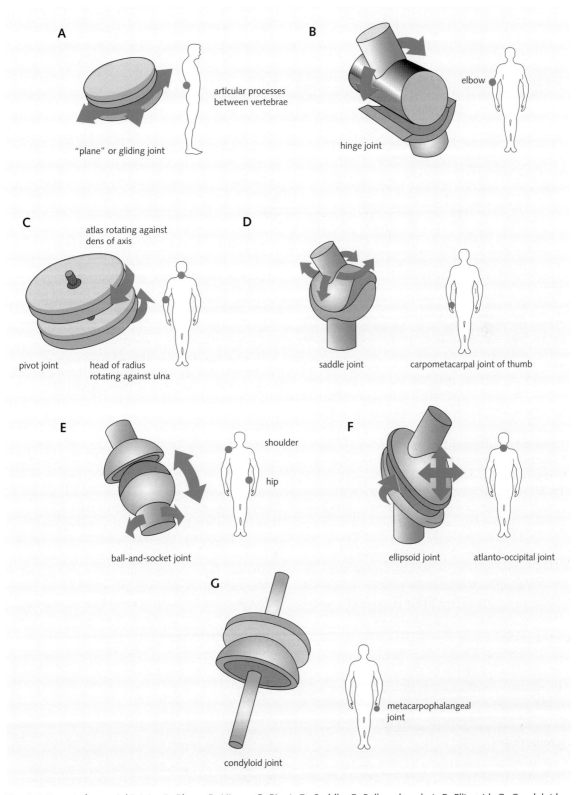

Fig. 5.5 Types of synovial joints. A. Plane. B. Hinge. C. Pivot. D. Saddle. E. Ball-and-socket. F. Ellipsoid. G. Condyloid.

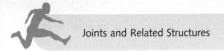
(i.e., biaxial movements). The metacarpophalangeal (MCP) and metatarsophalangeal (MTP) joints are examples of condyloid joints.

Blood supply and lymph drainage of joints

The periarticular arterial plexuses supply blood to the joints. These branch into articular arteries. They pierce the joint capsule to reach the synovium and communicate with one another to create rich anastomoses around and inside the joint.

Articular veins accompany the arteries, so they are also present in the joint capsule and synovial membrane. Lymphatic vessels are present in the synovial membrane and drain along the blood vessels to the regional lymph nodes.

Nerve supply of joints

Joints are richly supplied with articular nerves whose endings are located in both the fibrous capsule and synovial membrane. Articular nerves generally arise from the nerves supplying the muscles that move that particular joint. This is known as Hilton's law.

Both myelinated and nonmyelinated nerve fibers are present in articular nerves. They have different endings that correspond to their roles in sensory input. The main types of input are proprioception and pain.

Myelinated nerves have Ruffini endings, lamellated corpuscles (rather like pacinian corpuscles), and some resemble Golgi tendon organs. Both Ruffini endings and lancellated corpuscles register the speed and direction of movement, while Golgi organs, which are slower conducting, mediate joint position sense by providing information regarding the movement and position of the joint relative to the body. Nonmyelinated and finely myelinated nerves have free endings that are thought to mediate pain.

Arthropathies

Degenerative arthropathy
Osteoarthritis
Epidemiology
Osteoarthritis (OA) is the most common form of joint disorders. It first appears asymptomatically in the second and third decades of life and becomes almost universal by age 70. Almost all persons by age 40 have some osteoarthritic changes in weight-bearing joints, although relatively few are symptomatic. Men and women are equally affected, although onset is earlier in men. OA is particularly common in older adults, and although it occurs worldwide, it is less common in black populations.

Etiology
The etiology is essentially unknown. OA can be either primary or secondary. OA arising from no obvious cause (idiopathic) is known as primary OA. Predisposing factors include age (the condition is most common in older adults), genetic factors, biomechanical factors (e.g., lifestyle), and systemic factors such as obesity.

Secondary OA is less common than primary OA and tends to affect younger people. Causes include congenital abnormalities; genetics; trauma; occupational hazards (e.g., the knee joint in football players); avascular necrosis (e.g., sickle cell disease); and neuropathic, metabolic, endocrine, and other associated arthropathies or bone diseases.

There are several additional factors that predispose individuals to OA. These include family history, obesity, occupation (heavy physical work), age, and hypermobility.

Pathology
OA affects synovial joints, most commonly the distal interphalangeal (DIP) and first CMC joints in the hand (thumb), the MTP joints in the foot, the apophyseal (facet) joints of the spine, and weight-bearing joints such as the hip and knee.

In the early stages of OA, there is degeneration of cartilage (Fig. 5.6). This involves:
- Breakdown of cartilage caused by the release of enzymes from chondrocytes—the stimulus for this is unknown.
- Swelling and splitting of cartilage owing to the uptake of water. The loss of cartilage is variable, ranging from irregularity of the surface to full-thickness loss. This destruction leads to loss of joint space.
- Inflammation of synovium and joint capsule due to debris from the cartilage.

The inflammation associated with osteoarthritis is secondary to degeneration.

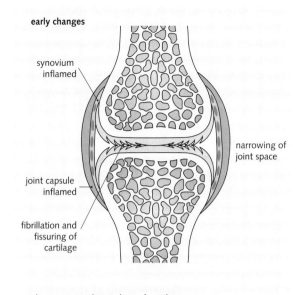

early changes

synovium inflamed

narrowing of joint space

joint capsule inflamed

fibrillation and fissuring of cartilage

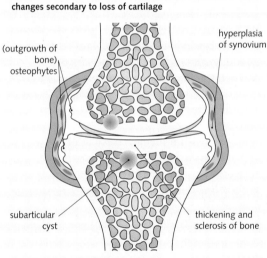

changes secondary to loss of cartilage

(outgrowth of bone) osteophytes

hyperplasia of synovium

subarticular cyst

thickening and sclerosis of bone

Fig. 5.6 Pathologic changes in osteoarthritis. The figure shows early changes and changes secondary to loss of cartilage.

In the later stages of OA, patients experience secondary changes in bone as a consequence of degeneration. This involves:

- Articulation of bone with bone because of cartilage loss, resulting in thickening and polishing (eburnation or sclerosis) of subarticular bone.
- Development of cysts in the newly sclerotic subarticular bone.
- Formation of osteophytes (overgrowth of bone) at articular margins.

- Hyperplasia of synovium due to inflammation.
- Development of deformity owing to loss of joint space.
- Immobility of a joint, resulting in disuse atrophy of muscle.

Clinical features

OA usually presents at around 50 years of age, although secondary OA may present earlier. Symptoms include:

- Intermittent or chronic pain at affected sites that is worse upon exertion (e.g., at the end of the day).
- Early morning stiffness that only lasts for a few minutes, in contrast to inflammatory arthritis in which stiffness lasts much longer.
- Pain in hands as well as the hips, knees, and spine (most commonly affected joints).

When only one joint is involved, there may be a history of previous pathology at that specific joint (i.e., injury). Signs include:

- Swelling at the affected joint due to effusion and osteophyte formation.
- Joint deformities with crepitus upon movement.
- Muscular wasting due to limited use of the joint.

In the hands, Heberden's nodes (swellings at the DIP) and Bouchard's nodes (swellings at the proximal interphalangeal joints [PIP]) may be present. There may also be "squaring" of the hand caused by changes at the thumb CMC joint.

At the hip, internal rotation is the first movement to be affected; passive movements also become painful at the end of the range of movement. There is also frequently a fixed flexion rotation (detected by Thomas test). Joints are usually affected bilaterally and symmetrically, although a unilateral pattern may be seen.

Diagnosis

OA is diagnosed clinically from the pattern of joints involved and the absence of systemic features. A plain X-ray demonstrates narrowing of the joint space and the presence of osteophytes, subchondral cysts, and osteosclerosis.

Blood tests are negative for rheumatoid factor and antinuclear antibodies (ANAs). Because OA is not a systemic disease, the erythrocyte sedimentation rate (ESR) is normal, and there is no evidence of anemia or abnormality of calcium metabolism. Analysis of synovial fluid shows an increase in volume and the

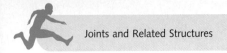

presence of white blood cells and crystals. Culture is negative.

Complications

OA has the potential to cause disability because of pain and decreased mobility.

Management

OA is treated by nonsteroidal anti-inflammatory drugs (NSAIDs) and analgesics to control pain; physicians should recommend that patients find a balance between exercise and rest and should advise patients on the progressive nature of the disease. Intra-articular steroids are occasionally used to reduce inflammation. Weight loss should be discussed if appropriate. Surgery may be needed to replace severely diseased joints.

Prognosis

OA is a progressive disease—affected joints slowly get worse, and other joints also become involved.

Inflammatory arthropathies
Rheumatoid arthritis: adult form

Rheumatoid arthritis is a systemic inflammatory disease that affects many parts of the body. It has a variable course, with periods of exacerbation and remission. Some patients have a self-limiting mild form of the condition, while the majority of patients experience a chronic destructive joint disease.

Epidemiology

Rheumatoid arthritis is polyarthritic, affecting at least 1% of Caucasians; the male:female ratio is 1:3. In adults, the peak of onset is between 25 and 50 years of age, although the disease can present at any age.

Etiology

The cause of rheumatoid arthritis is unknown; however, the condition is believed to involve an initiating factor that results in complex immunologic changes. There are a number of possible hypotheses.

Evidence supporting autoimmune mechanisms in rheumatoid arthritis includes:
• The presence of rheumatoid factor (an autoantibody).
• Circulating immune complexes—these are believed to be responsible for the extra-articular features.
• Defective T cell–mediated immunity.
• The presence of other autoimmune diseases.

Genetic factors are due to an association between human leukocyte antigen (HLA) DR4 and DR1. The initiating factor in rheumatoid arthritis has not been determined, although possible candidates include the Epstein–Barr virus and parvoviruses.

Pathology

The most common sites affected in rheumatoid arthritis are the small joints of the hands (especially the PIP and MCP joints, as opposed to the DIP joints in OA). The wrist, elbow, shoulder, cervical spine, hip, and knee may also become involved. Note that secondary changes include muscle wasting and osteoporosis.

The disease process can be split into three stages (Fig. 5.7). These include:
• Inflammation of the synovium—there is an infiltration of lymphocytes and macrophages.
• Destruction of cartilage—pannus (a layer of chronically inflamed fibrous tissue) extends across the cartilage, destroying it.
• Destruction of bone due to pannus—this results in joint deformities (e.g., ulnar deviation, swan-neck, and boutonnière deformities in the hand).

Clinical features

Symptoms include:
• Joint pain with prolonged early morning stiffness and "gelling" of the joint after activity.
• Fatigue and general malaise.
• Weight loss during active disease.
• Anemia.
• Extra-articular symptoms (Fig. 5.8).

Signs include:
• Warm and tender joints, with insidious onset, first affecting the small joints of the hands and feet and then progressing to other joints.
• Swelling.
• Subcutaneous rheumatoid nodules.
• Decreased movement.

In the later stages, the joint deformities mentioned previously and muscle wasting may be seen. Splenomegaly and lymphadenopathy may be present. The joints are affected symmetrically, and the disease is progressive with remissions.

Diagnosis

The diagnosis of rheumatoid arthritis is made clinically from the pattern of joints involved, the presence of rheumatoid nodules, and episodes of remission.

inflammation of synovium

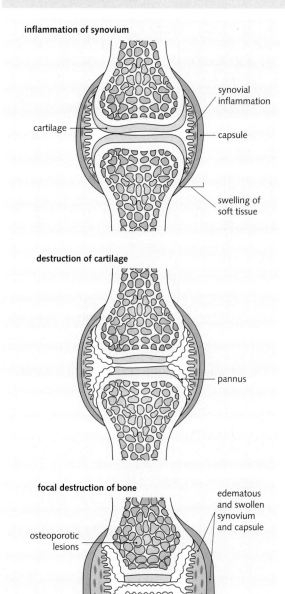

synovial inflammation

cartilage

capsule

swelling of soft tissue

destruction of cartilage

pannus

focal destruction of bone

edematous and swollen synovium and capsule

osteoporotic lesions

erosion of the bone leading to joint deformity

Fig. 5.7 Pathologic changes in rheumatoid arthritis. These changes include inflammation of synovium, destruction of cartilage, and focal destruction of bone.

About 70–80% of patients have rheumatoid factor present, and about 30% have ANAs. The ESR and C-reactive protein levels are raised, and patients may have an associated anemia and thrombocytosis.

A plain X-ray will demonstrate narrowing of joint spaces with the presence of subchondral cysts. In addition, osteoporosis may be present in bone adjacent to the affected joint and focal erosions of bone. Synovial fluid is usually turbid and green/yellow in color. White blood cells are present, and culture is negative.

Complications
Rheumatoid arthritis can cause secondary OA and/or septic arthritis.

Rheumatoid arthritis can also be severely disabling.

Management
Rheumatoid arthritis is treated with NSAIDs to control pain and immunosuppressive drugs, such as penicillamine, methotrexate, gold, and corticosteroids. Side effects of drug treatment include gastrointestinal bleeding and renal impairment. Patient education and physiotherapy are also important aspects of management. Treatment is aimed at controlling the symptoms and at modifying disease activity rather than eradicating the cause.

Rheumatoid arthritis: juvenile form
The juvenile form of rheumatoid arthritis presents in individuals before the age of 16 years; the prognosis is worse than in adults.

Sjögren's syndrome
Affecting the exocrine glands, Sjögren's syndrome is a chronic inflammatory disease of unknown etiology that is either primary or secondary to connective tissue diseases. It is also associated with rheumatic disorders, the most common of which is rheumatoid arthritis, but the list also includes systemic lupus erythematosus, scleroderma, polymyositis, and juvenile rheumatoid arthritis.

The lymphatic infiltration of exocrine glands leads to keratoconjunctivitis sicca (dry eyes) and xerostomia (dry mouth). The condition is treated symptomatically by use of artificial tears and pilocarpine hydrochloride tablets, which increase secretion from the salivary glands.

Seronegative arthritides
The seronegative arthritides are a group of related disorders. They are similar because they:
- Are often associated with HLA B27 (human leukocyte antigen B27).
- Are negative for rheumatoid factor and other autoantibodies.
- Have a familial tendency.
- Are more common in caucasian people.

Extra-articular features of rheumatoid disease	
Site	Manifestation
Nerves	Carpal tunnel syndrome, peripheral neuropathy ('glove and stocking' sensory loss)
Skin	Subcutaneous nodules (particularly on extensor aspect of forearm near elbow), vasculitic lesions
Blood vessels	Vasculitis
Eyes	Episcleritis, scleritis, secondary Sjögren's syndrome (i.e. triad of dry mouth, dry eyes, and arthritis)
Chest	Intrapulmonary nodules, pleural effusions, fibrosing alveolitis, Caplan's syndrome
Heart	Myocarditis, pericarditis, pericardial effusion
Kidney	Amyloidosis, impaired renal function may be side effect of drug treatment
Soft tissues around joints	Bursitis, tenosynovitis

Fig. 5.8 Extra-articular features of rheumatoid disease.

Patients may present with several different disorders, occurring either simultaneously or at different times.

Ankylosing spondylitis

Ankylosing spondylitis is the most common cause of inflammatory neck and back pain in young adults (Fig. 5.9). It is primarily characterized by inflammation of the axial skeleton and large peripheral joints.

Epidemiology

The male:female ratio in ankylosing spondylitis is estimated to be of the order of 2–3:1. Women tend to show milder symptoms. Onset is usually in young adults.

Etiology

There is a familial tendency in acquiring ankylosing spondylitis, with the HLA B27 association occurring in 90% of affected individuals.

Pathology

The spinal (vertebral) joints are affected in patients with ankylosing spondylitis. Inflammation starts in the lumbar spine and sacroiliac joints and extends proximally. The pathology begins at sites of ligamentous insertions, resulting in enthesopathy (inflammation at tendinous insertion into bone)—the hallmark of spondyloarthropathies.

There are initial erosive lesions on the vertebral body that lead to the growth of bony spurs across the annulus fibrosis, called syndesmophytes. The upper and lower syndesmophytes across each intervertebral disc fuse together, thus fusing the spine. On X-rays, there is "squaring" of the vertebral bodies, and the appearance of the fused spine gives rise to the "bamboo spine" tag.

Clinical features

Most patients with ankylosing spondylitis present in their late teens or early adulthood.

Symptoms include:
- Back pain, pelvic pain, and joint pain in the lower limbs.
- Systemic manifestations, including iritis and aortic valve incompetence.

Signs that may be present include:
- Kyphosis.
- Limited spinal flexion.
- Decreased chest expansion.

Diagnosis

Ankylosing spondylitis is diagnosed by the presence of HLA B27 (90%), although unaffected individuals may also carry this antigen (16%). ESR and C-reactive protein levels are often elevated. A spinal radiograph may demonstrate calcification and ossification, the so-called tramline or bamboo spine appearance.

Management

Ankylosing spondylitis is usually treated with NSAIDs, immunosuppressive drugs such as sulphasalazine, and regular exercise to maintain

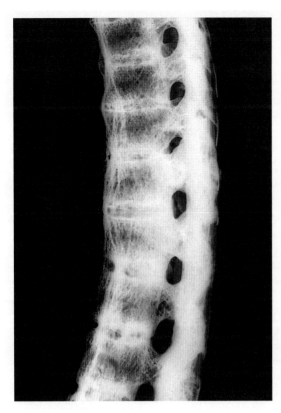

Fig. 5.9 Radiograph of a sagittal section through the vertebral column showing ankylosing spondylitis. There is complete fusion of the spine and apophyseal joints, and fusion also occurs across the intervertebral disc (courtesy of Dr PG Bullough).

movement; hip replacement is occasionally required if the hip is ankylosed (fused).

Prognosis

Although ankylosing spondylitis is progressive, most patients are able to lead a normal life.

Arthritis associated with gastrointestinal disease
Enteropathic arthritis

Enteropathic arthritis is associated with inflammatory bowel disease (IBD): ulcerative colitis or Crohn's disease. The severity of the arthritis, which affects the knees, ankles, and elbows, reflects the activity of the IBD, with most episodes resolving within a few months. Successful treatment of the IBD usually leads to remission of enteropathic arthritis. Most episodes resolve within a few months.

Arthritis associated with other systemic diseases
Reactive arthritis

Reactive arthritis occurs in response to infection at a distant site, unlike septic arthritis, which is characterized by the ability to isolate organisms from the joint itself. The main causative organisms are:

- *Chlamydia*, causing a genital infection.
- *Salmonella*, *Campylobacter*, or *Shigella*, causing a gastrointestinal infection.

Reactive arthritis is more common in males and is the most common cause of arthritis in young males. About 80% of patients show an association with HLA B27, suggesting an autoimmune process. Reactive arthritis is often termed Reiter's syndrome when it follows a diarrheal or sexually transmitted infection and is characterized by a triad of arthritis, urethritis/cervicitis, and conjunctivitis. The arthritis usually affects the knees or ankles (asymmetrical oligoarthritis), although axial disease may occur.

The changes seen histologically are similar to those of rheumatoid arthritis, and the diagnosis is clinical. Although symptoms may clear spontaneously, a large number of patients will suffer recurrences. In a minority, severe spondylitis may develop. In patients who are HIV-positive, a very severe form of reactive arthritis may result.

Psoriatic arthritis

Psoriatic arthritis occurs in 5–10% of psoriasis sufferers. It may also occur in individuals with a family history of psoriasis. HLA B27 association is often seen if spondylitis is also present. Psoriatic arthritis may be clinically indistinguishable from rheumatoid arthritis, with the DIP joints most affected; axial involvement may also occur. Radiography may show bone erosion and periarticular osteoporosis.

Treatment is with NSAIDs and analgesics. Immunosuppressive drugs may also be used. In a minority of cases, severe destruction of bone may occur (i.e., arthritis mutilans).

Behçet's syndrome

Behçet's syndrome is a rare condition of unknown etiology. Cases are most commonly found in Japan and around the Mediterranean. The main features are

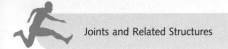

polyarthritis, iritis, and oral/genital ulceration. Less commonly, a patient may experience neurologic, skin, or gastrointestinal symptoms. The condition is characterized by exacerbations and remissions and is treated with administration of oral steroids.

Still's disease

Still's disease is the most common cause of chronic juvenile arthritis (i.e., arthritis occurring in a person under 16 years of age). Some forms of Still's disease are similar to rheumatoid arthritis. Systemic symptoms include a salmon-colored rash, spiking fever, lymphadenopathy, splenomegaly, and pericarditis. The number of joints affected is variable, depending on the subtype of Still's disease. Most patients recover spontaneously before early adulthood.

Sarcoid arthritis

Sarcoid arthritis is a transient polyarthritis or an acute monoarthritis that occurs in patients with sarcoidosis. An acute arthritis is commonly a presenting feature of sarcoidosis and is often accompanied by erythema nodosum and hilar lymphadenopathy. The sites affected are usually large joints, such as ankles and knees. Sarcoidosis, which presents with arthritis, has a good prognosis and is usually self-remitting.

Neuropathic joint disease (Charcot's joint)

In neuropathic joint disease, or Charcot's joint, loss of sensation results in traumatic joint damage. The conditions associated with Charcot's joint are as follows:

* Diabetes mellitus—joints in the feet are affected.
* Tabes dorsalis following syphilis—ankle and knee joints are affected.
* Leprosy—joint affected varies according to the site of sensory loss.

Arthritis associated with hemodialysis

Arthritis can arise as a result of hemodialysis; the condition is caused by the deposition of amyloid in the joints and periarticular tissues. Oxalate crystal deposition may occur in chronic renal disorders.

Systemic lupus erythematosus

Systemic lupus erythematosus (SLE) is a connective tissue disorder usually presenting with joint symptoms that resemble those of rheumatoid arthritis.

Crystal arthropathies

The crystal arthropathies are a group of disorders in which the deposition of crystals in joints leads to inflammation.

Gout
Epidemiology

Gout is more common in men, although some postmenopausal women may be affected.

Etiology

In patients with gout, hyperuricemia results in the deposition of monosodium urate crystals in the joint. In patients with primary gout, the causes of hyperuricemia are commonly idiopathic, usually because of impaired excretion. There is a familial tendency in acquiring gout. Secondary gout may occur as a result of:

* Increased production of uric acid (e.g., increased cell turnover in carcinomas and leukemia following chemotherapy).
* Enzyme defects.
* Impaired excretion (e.g., renal failure).
* Alcohol consumption.
* Hyperlipidemia.
* High purine intake in the diet.

Pathology

Uric acid is a product of DNA (purine) breakdown and is normally excreted in the urine. Excess uric acid results in the deposition of crystals in:

* Joints—the most commonly affected being the MTP joint in the big toe. The ankle joint may also be affected.
* Soft tissues—this may lead to the formation of tophi (palpable masses).
* The urinary tract, in the form of urate stones.

The deposition of crystals in the synovium and periarticular soft tissues causes an acute inflammatory reaction, which may be precipitated by alcohol, diet, surgery, or drugs. Chronic gouty arthritis occurs following recurrent attacks. This condition is characterized by cartilage degeneration, synovial hyperplasia, and secondary OA.

Clinical features

Patients with gout present between the ages of 20 and 60 years, although most commonly they present in middle age. An acute attack involves an extremely painful monoarthritis of sudden onset. The affected joint is edematous and red; more than one joint may be affected in certain cases.

Diagnosis

The presence of tophi on the earlobes or around joints may aid in the diagnosis of gout. Microscopy of synovial fluid demonstrates the presence of needle-shaped crystals that are diagnostic. These crystals are negatively birefringent. Neutrophils are also found. Plasma uric acid levels are raised at >0.5 mmol/L, and there are also raised ESR levels and a raised white cell count.

Complications

Renal disease is a complication of gout. Hyperuricemia is genetically associated with an increased risk of hypertension and coronary artery disease.

Management

An acute attack of gout is treated with NSAIDs and aspiration of joint effusions.

Allopurinol, a drug that decreases uric acid synthesis, is used in the long term. The patient should be advised to maintain good fluid intake and avoid precipitating factors.

Prognosis

Attacks of gout may be infrequent, and treatment can reduce the extent of joint damage. However, renal complications are frequent.

Pseudogout

Pseudogout is a condition that may mimic gout. It is more common in older adults. In patients with pseudogout, calcium pyrophosphate crystals are deposited in the articular cartilage. Inflammation results if the crystals are shed into the joint space.

When pseudogout occurs in people younger than 60 years of age, it is often associated with hyperparathyroidism and hemochromatosis. The joints most commonly affected are the knee, wrist, shoulder, and ankle. Pseudogout can be differentiated from gout by the presence of brick-shaped crystals in the synovial fluid that are positively birefringent.

Arthritis associated with infection
Septic arthritis
Epidemiology

Infectious (septic) arthritis is an uncommon condition, usually affecting children and young adults. Acute bacterial arthritis is a medical emergency.

Etiology

Infectious arthritis is usually caused by bacteria such as *Staphylococcus aureus*, *Streptococcus pyogenes*, *Neisseria gonorrhoeae*, *Haemophilus influenzae*, and gram-negative organisms. Tuberculous arthritis is now relatively rare. A viral cause, such as rubella or mumps, is less common for infectious arthritis.

There are several predisposing factors. These include:
- Prosthetic joints.
- Drug addiction.
- Age between 5 and 15 years.
- Diabetes mellitus.
- Immunosuppressive drugs.
- Rheumatoid arthritis.

Pathology

In patients with infectious arthritis, the infecting organism gains access to the joint:
- Hematogenously.
- As a result of local trauma.
- By direct spread from adjacent foci of infection.

Clinical features

Only one joint is usually affected in infectious arthritis; the patient typically presents with a painful and swollen erythematous joint and an associated fever. Very little movement is possible at the joint, and there are systemic signs of sepsis. The joint should be aspirated for culture if infection is suspected. Septic arthritis must be excluded in children who present with a painful joint because the disease causes devastating damage to the joint if left undiagnosed.

Diagnosis

Synovial fluid is turbid in infectious arthritis, and white blood cells are present. Culture is positive. Patients need an X-ray to exclude trauma.

Management

Intravenous antibiotic treatment should be started immediately if infectious arthritis is diagnosed. This is initially "blind" until the culture results are available. Treatment with oral antibiotics is continued for 6 weeks, and for at least 2 weeks after all signs and symptoms of inflammation have subsided. Drainage of the joint is needed to remove debris. The joint should also be immobilized.

Prognosis

Infectious arthritis can be life threatening; hence, it is important to get immediate treatment. Recovery can take from a few days to a few weeks.

Disorders affecting specific joints

Disorders of the hand and wrist
Osteoarthritis of the wrist and hand
The joints of the hand are commonly affected by OA. The CMC joint of the thumb feels tender, and there is limited abduction.

Etiology
The etiology is unknown. OA appears to be the result of a complete system of interacting, predisposing factors, including congenital, genetic, environmental, metabolic, and neuropathic factors.

Clinical Features
In patients with OA of the wrist and hand, the interphalangeal joints become painful and stiff, with osteophytes creating swellings; these are called Heberden's nodes at the DIP and Bouchard's nodes at the PIP joints. The wrists are usually affected at a later stage after trauma (lower radius or scaphoid fracture).

Rheumatoid arthritis of the wrist and hand
Complications
The wrists and hands usually suffer a major loss of function and deformities in rheumatoid arthritis.

Progressively, there is synovitis of the proximal joints and tendon sheaths; then erosions occur, and, finally, joint derangement and tendon rupture lead to structural and functional losses.

The fingers have swan-neck (hyperextended PIP joint and flexed DIP joint) or boutonnière (flexed PIP joint, hyperextended DIP joint, and extended MCP joint) deformities (Fig. 5.10).

The thumb acquires a Z deformity. The MCP joints and wrists undergo subluxation so that the fingers show ulnar deviation. The ulnar styloid and radial head become prominent. There may also be firm rheumatoid nodules on the extensor surfaces and the flexor tendons.

de Quervain's tenosynovitis
de Quervain's tenosynovitis is inflammation of the fibrous sheath containing the tendons of extensor pollicis brevis and abductor pollicis longus muscles. The tendons and the sheath become inflamed as they pass over the styloid process of the radius. Pain is felt at the styloid process of the radius; swelling of the tendon occurs, and a there is also a palpable nodule proximal to the wrist joint on the radial aspect.

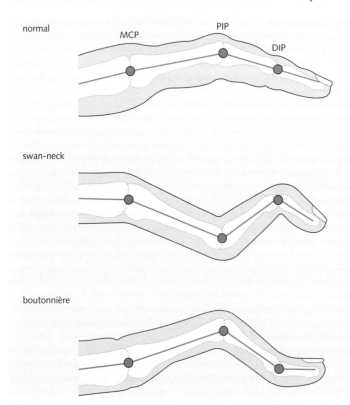

normal
MCP
PIP
DIP

swan-neck

boutonnière

Fig. 5.10 Finger deformities in rheumatoid arthritis: normal finger, swan-neck, and boutonnière deformities.

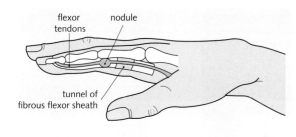

flexor tendons nodule

tunnel of fibrous flexor sheath

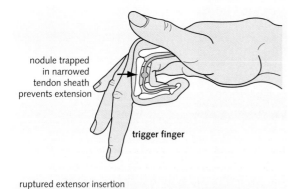

nodule trapped in narrowed tendon sheath prevents extension

trigger finger

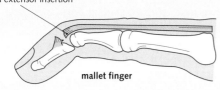

ruptured extensor insertion

mallet finger

Fig. 5.11 "Trigger finger" and "mallet finger" due to tendon injuries. See text for details.

de Quervain's tenosynovitis may be caused by overuse of the tendons (e.g., wringing out, washing). Treatment of de Quervain's tenosynovitis is by hydrocortisone injection or surgically splitting the tendon sheath.

Tendon lesions
Trigger finger
"Trigger finger," or digital stenosing synovitis, is a thickening of the tendon sheaths that constricts the flexor tendons (Fig. 5.11). This condition affects the ring and middle fingers in adults and the thumb in children. Extension of the finger has to be forced through a narrower space and elicits a snap noise. It is treated with steroid injections.

Mallet finger
"Mallet finger" is also called "baseball finger" (see Fig. 5.11). The extensor tendon is damaged at its insertion into the distal phalanx so that the DIP joint cannot be fully extended. It is treated by splinting the finger with the DIP joint fully extended.

Dropped finger
"Dropped finger" is caused by tendon rupture at the wrist—either direct or as a complication of rheumatoid arthritis—resulting in loss of finger extension at the MCP joint.

Ganglia
Ganglia are smooth cystic swellings containing clear viscous fluid rich in mucopolysaccharides, and they appear as painless lumps usually on the dorsum of the wrist (Fig. 5.12). They are mostly unilocular and have

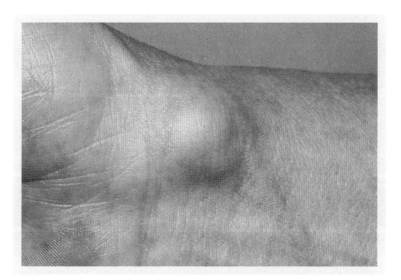

Fig. 5.12 Ganglion at the dorsal surface of the wrist (courtesy of Dr. JH Klippel).

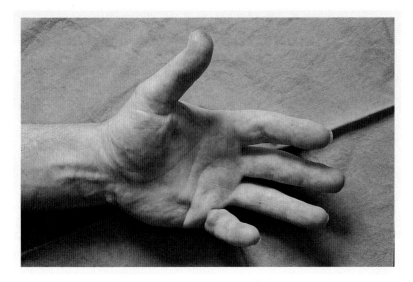

Fig. 5.13 Dupuytren's contracture of the palmar fascia (courtesy of Dr. JH Klippel).

capsules of fibrous tissue. Ganglia form around the joint capsule and tendon sheath, to which they are attached, but they do not usually communicate with the joint space. Ganglia are treated by excision only if they press on the local ulnar or median nerves.

Dupuytren's contracture
Etiology
In Dupuytren's contracture, the palmar aponeurosis is thickened and contracted, and there is skin tethering (Fig. 5.13). Dupuytren's contracture is commonly bilateral, symmetrical, and painless. The fingers become flexed at the MCP and PIP joints. There may be fibrous thickenings in the dorsal knuckle pads (Garod's pads) and on the soles of the feet. The precise etiology of the condition is unknown, although it is thought to be associated with microtrauma.

Epidemiology
Dupuytren's contracture affects more men than women; may be familial; and has associations with alcoholism, antiepileptic drugs, and Peyronie's disease (fibrosis of the corpus cavernosum).

Management
Dupuytren's contracture is treated by surgical excision of the thickened region but only when the deformity is progressive.

Carpal tunnel syndrome
Etiology
Carpal tunnel syndrome is caused by median nerve compression as it passes under the flexor retinaculum at the wrist. The syndrome usually occurs following a repetitive stress injury to the wrist, such as that caused by hammering, typing, and other such activities. It is a type of compartment syndrome and occurs in premenstrual and pregnant women, in cases of myxedema and rheumatoid arthritis, as well as in patients with severe burns.

Clinical features
Carpal tunnel syndrome is associated with paresthesia and pain in the median nerve distribution in the hand (thumb, index, and middle and radial half of the ring finger). Pain is worse at night and after repetitive movements. Later symptoms include wasting and decreased sensation of the thenar eminence.

Management
Carpal tunnel syndrome is treated either conservatively with diuretics and hydrocortisone injections or by surgical (open or arthroscopic) division of the flexor retinaculum.

Disorders of the elbow
Tennis elbow
Tennis elbow is inflammation of the common extensor attachment at the lateral epicondyle (lateral epicondylitis) and causes pain and disability.

Etiology
Tennis elbow may be caused by excessive, repetitive, and strenuous overuse of the wrist and digit extensors and pronator, such as during backhand tennis or squash, manual screwdriving, or other such activities.

Management

Tennis elbow is treated with physical therapy, rest, avoidance of the offending activity, or steroid injections. Surgical release of the extensor origin may become necessary if conservative approaches fail.

Golfer's elbow

Golfer's elbow is inflammation of the common flexor attachment at the medial epicondyle (medial epicondylitis).

Etiology

Golfer's elbow may occur due to excessive, strenuous overuse of the wrist and digit flexors, such as during opening tight jars, playing forehand tennis, and golfing.

Management

Golfer's elbow is treated with physical therapy, rest, avoidance of the offending maneuvers, or steroid injections. During infection and if surgical release is necessary, the proximity of the ulnar nerve to the medical epicondyle should be noted.

Olecranon bursitis

Olecranon bursitis occurs after trauma, sepsis, rheumatoid arthritis, and gout. It involves a hot, painful swelling behind the olecranon process. Traumatic bursitis is also referred to as "student's elbow"—caused by propping of the elbows on desks for long periods, as in studying. If infection is suspected, the joint must be aspirated.

Cubitus valgus and cubitus varus

Cubitus valgus is when the "carrying angle" of the elbow joint is greater than the normal 10 degrees in men and 15 degrees in women (Fig. 5.14). The condition is caused by malunion of a previous lateral condylar fracture or retarded lateral epiphyseal growth. There may be an association with Turner's syndrome. Complications include ulnar neuritis and OA.

Cubitus varus is the opposite deformity, with a decreased carrying angle (see Fig. 5.14). Its most common cause is malunion of a supracondylar fracture. Cubitus valgus and cubitus varus may be corrected by osteotomy.

Ulnar neuritis
Etiology

In patients with ulnar neuritis, the ulnar nerve may be subjected to constriction (OA, rheumatoid arthritis) because constant friction (cubitus valgus), because it lies in a groove behind the medial epicondyle. This

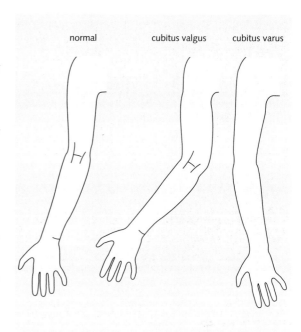

normal   cubitus valgus   cubitus varus

Fig. 5.14 Normal angle of the elbow, cubitus valgus, and cubitus varus.

can lead to nerve fibrosis and eventual ulnar neuropathy. The condition may also be involved in leprosy and fractures of the medial epicondyle.

Complications

Ulnar neuritis is characterized by hand clumsiness, reduced sensation over the little finger and the medial side of the ring finger, and weakened intrinsic muscles of the hand innervated by the ulnar nerve.

Management

Treatment of ulnar neuritis involves surgery for nerve release and transposition of the nerve to the front of the elbow.

Loose bodies in the elbow joint

Loose bodies in the elbow joint may arise from osteochondral fractures, osteophytes of OA, and other conditions, such as synovial chondromatosis and osteochondritis dissecans. They cause locking of the elbow as the bodies become stuck between the bones, causing sharp pain and swelling, and are treated by surgical removal.

Rheumatoid arthritis of the elbow

For more than half of all patients with rheumatoid arthritis, the elbow joint is affected by the condition. Patients experience pain and limitation of movement in both the elbow and superior radiohumeral joints.

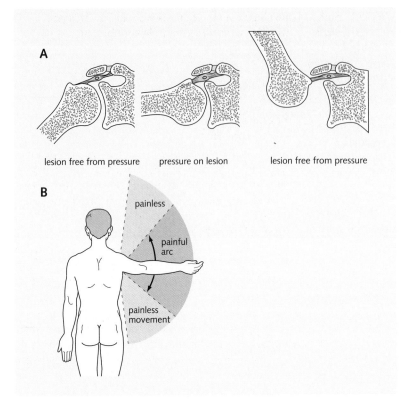

lesion free from pressure   pressure on lesion   lesion free from pressure

painless

painful
arc

painless
movement

Fig. 5.15 Mechanism and etiology
of painful arc syndrome.
A. Mechanical basis. B. Areas
of pain.

The joint is treated conservatively; removal of the
synovium or joint replacement may also be considered.

Disorders of the shoulder
Dislocation of the shoulder joint
A dislocated shoulder joint is a very common injury,
usually caused by falling onto an outstretched arm
(e.g., when playing rugby or football). The joint may
be displaced in different directions, but anterior
displacement of the humeral head to below the
coracoid process is the most common occurrence
(anterior dislocation, subcoracoid dislocation).

Complications
Complications of a dislocated shoulder include neural
(axillary nerve) and arterial (posterior circumflex
humeral artery) damage, joint stiffness, and recurrent
dislocations. Axillary nerve involvement is usually
diagnosed by demonstrating a patch of anesthesia on
the skin over the lateral aspect of the deltoid muscle,
which is supplied by the upper lateral cutaneous branch
of this nerve.

Management
A dislocated shoulder is treated by reducing the
joint and immobilizing it for about 3 weeks.

Painful arc syndrome
In painful arc syndrome, shoulder abduction causes
pain in the midranges but not during extremes of
movement (i.e., between 45 and 150 degrees).
Degeneration is the underlying defect, and pain is
caused by impingement of an inflamed structure
between the greater tuberosity and the acromion
(Fig. 5.15).

Etiology
Painful arc syndrome may be caused by incomplete
tearing of the supraspinatus tendon, supraspinatus
tendinitis, subacromial bursitis, and fracture of the
greater tuberosity of the humerus. The lesions may
be associated with supraspinatus tendon calcification
(perhaps a variation of crystal arthropathy),
rheumatoid arthritis, or acromioclavicular joint OA.

Management
Painful arc syndrome is treated with steroid
injections and surgery.

Rotator cuff tears
Rotator cuff tears are partial tears that often occur
with supraspinatus tendinitis, leading to painful arc
syndrome and pain on moving the arm forcibly

forward. Complete tears limit shoulder abduction, cause joint pain at the shoulder tip and upper arm, and tenderness under the acromion. The tears are usually in the supraspinatus tendon, although subscapularis and infraspinatus may be involved. Chronic irritation may lead to subacromial bursitis.

Etiology
Rotator cuff tears may be caused by athletic injuries (e.g., baseball pitchers, freestyle swimmers, violent throwing activities) or by age-related degeneration or a fall (e.g., in epileptic subjects).

Management
Rotator cuff tears are treated by repairing the tendon; better results are obtained in young people with less degeneration.

Adhesive capsulitis (frozen shoulder)
Adhesive capsulitis or "frozen shoulder" is a common but poorly understood condition affecting the glenohumeral joint. It causes pain and limitation of all movements (to about half the normal range), but no changes are seen on an X-ray.

Etiology
Adhesive capsulitis may follow a minor injury or may be due to an autoimmune response to localized rotator cuff tissues. Recovery usually follows the course of pain, stiffness, and recuperation phases. It may take months to heal.

Management
Adhesive capsulitis is treated initially with NSAIDs, analgesics, and gentle exercise. Joint manipulation is undertaken when the joint is stronger.

Biceps rupture
In biceps rupture, an aching in the shoulder often occurs after "something snaps" during lifting. A "ball" appears in the muscle belly on elbow flexion.

Etiology
Biceps rupture may be caused by athletic injuries or degenerative changes or a fall.

Management
Because the function of the biceps remains intact during rupture, no treatment is required.

Biceps tendinitis
Biceps tendinitis is an uncommon condition, but rotator cuff tears may involve the long head of biceps,

causing pain in the anterior shoulder. This pain worsens with forced muscle contraction.

Management
Biceps tendinitis is treated by physical therapy and steroid injection.

Rheumatoid arthritis and osteoarthritis in the shoulder
Rheumatoid arthritis and OA are not as common in the shoulder as they are in weight-bearing hip and knee joints. Pain and restricted movement are treated by analgesics and ultimately by joint replacement.

Pain referred to the shoulder
Pain referred to the shoulder may occur via C5 to the deltoid; C6, C7, and C8 to the superior border of the scapula; or C3 and C4 from the diaphragm to the shoulder tip.

The brachial plexus and roots (e.g., prolapsed cervical disc, herpes zoster, cervical rib), upper arm, abdomen (e.g., cholecystitis, subphrenic abscess), and thorax (e.g., angina, pleurisy) may contribute to referred pain.

Disorders of the hip
Coxa vara
Etiology
Coxa vara includes any condition in which the angle between the neck and the shaft of the femur is less than the normal 125 degrees (Fig. 5.16). This leads to true shortening of the limb and a limping walk due to a Trendelenburg "dip."

The cause of coxa vara may be:
- Congenital.
- A slipped upper femoral epiphysis.
- Fracture (trochanteric with malunion, nonunited fractures of the femoral neck).
- Bone softening (rickets, osteomalacia, or Paget's disease of bone).

Congenital dislocation of the hip
Epidemiology
Congenital dislocation of the hip (CDH) should be diagnosed and corrected in the first week of life to prevent delayed walking and abnormal gait. Girls are eight times more likely to have CDH than boys, with the left hip more commonly involved than the right. The condition occurs more frequently after a breech delivery and if a relative is affected. The acetabulum is abnormally shallow with a very superiorly sloping

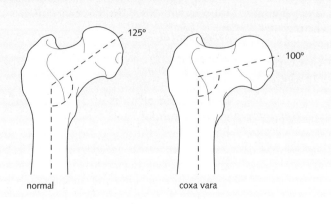

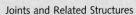

Fig. 5.16 Normal femur and coxa vara.

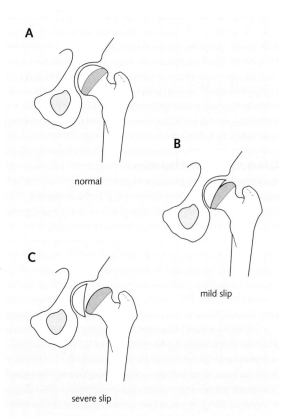

Fig. 5.17 Types of epiphysis. A. Normal femoral epiphysis. B. Mild case. C. Severely slipped upper femoral epiphysis.

roof, the femoral head is displaced upward and laterally, and the joint capsule may fold inward.

Management
CDH is treated in various ways according to the age of the patient. Treatment may involve splints, joint reduction, osteotomy, or hip displacement.

Perthes' disease
Perthes' disease occurs in children and involves osteochondritis of the epiphysis of the femoral head. There is avascular necrosis of unknown cause, resulting in bone fragmentation with concurrent revascularization and new bone formation. Narrowing of the joint space and flattening of the femoral head occur, and these are risks for early arthritis. Surgical containment is necessary to treat severe cases of Perthes' disease.

Slipped upper femoral epiphysis
Etiology
In adolescents, there may be a displacement of the upper epiphysis downward and backward from the femoral neck along the epiphyseal line (Fig. 5.17). This slipped upper femoral epiphysis affects overweight patients and males more than females. The patient experiences limping; pain in the groin, thigh, or knee; and limited abduction. Complications include avascular necrosis of the femoral head and coxa vara.

Management
A slipped upper femoral epiphysis is treated by pinning the femur into position and performing an osteotomy.

Transient synovitis
Transient synovitis is a short-lived condition of childhood and is of unknown etiology. It causes pain, limping, and limited hip movements. X-rays are normal. No treatment is required for transient synovitis because the patient recovers spontaneously in about 4 weeks.

Tuberculous arthritis
Etiology
Tuberculosis (TB) frequently affects the hip joint, causing pain, limping, limited movement, and muscle spasm. X-rays show bone rarefaction (decreased density but normal volume) and subsequent articular cartilage and bony erosion.

Management
Tuberculous arthritis is treated with antituberculous drugs. If the joint has been destroyed, arthrodesis (joint fusion) is performed.

Osteoarthritis of the hip
Etiology
OA of the hip is a very common cause of disability, especially in older adults. It may develop from general wear and tear or as a sequel to acetabular injuries, Perthes' disease, coxa vara, or slipped femoral epiphysis.

Pathology
In patients with OA of the hip, the articular cartilage is worn away where stress is transmitted. The underlying bone becomes sclerotic, and there is cyst formation; the patient may also have synovial hypertrophy, capsular fibrosis, and osteophytes in the joint margins. Pain occurs in the groin and may also radiate to the knee; pain worsens with walking and is relieved by rest. All hip movements are limited.

Management
The treatment of OA of the hip depends on its severity. Treatment is either conservative (i.e., with administration of analgesics and hydrocortisone injections) or surgical, by osteotomy, joint replacement, or arthrodesis.

Rheumatoid arthritis of the hip
The hip is frequently affected in rheumatoid arthritis. The patient experiences progressive femoral head erosion that leads to leg shortening, limited movement, gluteal and thigh muscle wasting, and gradual pain. Rheumatoid arthritis is treated conservatively with NSAIDs and immunosuppressants or by hip replacement.

Pain referred to the hip
Pain may be referred to the hip from the knee, spine (prolapsed disc, sacroiliac arthritis), the pelvis and lower abdomen (appendicular abscess, pyosalpinx,

irritation of the obturator nerve or muscle spasm), or from thrombosis of the lower abdominal aorta and its main branches.

Abnormal gait
Etiology
Abnormal gait may arise when there is a loss of coordination in the movements of the spine, hip, knee, ankle, and foot.

There are several types of abnormal gait, including:
- Osteogenic gait—bone shortening leads to limping.
- Arthrogenic gait—ankylosis; fixed flexion deformity, making one or both buttocks prominent, and abduction deformity, where the lower limb in the swing phase swings around the lower limb in the stance phase (on the ground) during gait.
- Myogenic gait—weak gluteal muscles in muscular dystrophy, causing a waddling gait.
- Neurogenic gait—disorders such as hemiparesis, cerebellar ataxia, parkinsonism, cerebral palsy, footdrop, and bilateral leg spasticity all show characteristic gaits.

Disorders of the knee
Genu varum and genu valgum
Genu varum (bow legs) and genu valgum (knock knees) commonly occur in childhood and usually correct spontaneously (Fig. 5.18). They may also

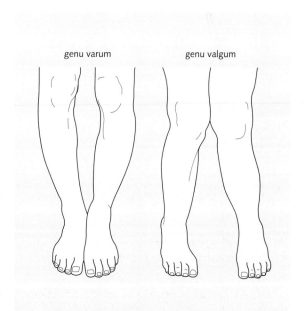

Fig. 5.18 Genu varum and genu valgum.

occur secondary to injury or disease (fractures, rheumatoid arthritis or OA, rickets, osteomalacia, and Paget's disease of bone).

Meniscal tears

Epidemiology
Meniscal tears are common in young men. They are usually caused by a twisting injury, typically while playing sports.

Etiology
The medial meniscus is torn more often than the lateral meniscus, since it is less mobile. When the meniscus splits longitudinally, a "bucket-handle" tear occurs in which the meniscus remains attached at both ends; if either end becomes detached, anterior horn or posterior horn tears are produced (Fig. 5.19). The torn meniscal tags may either cause mechanical "locking" of the knee by becoming jammed between the tibia and femur (preventing full extension) or predispose the individual to secondary OA because of the irritation to the joint.

Management
Meniscal tears are treated by arthroscopic excision of the torn or displaced tag.

Tears of the cruciate ligament
Severe injuries to the knee during skiing or other sports (especially football and hockey) that involve forced abduction, external rotation, and semiflexion of the knee may result in tears of the anterior cruciate ligament.

Tears of the posterior cruciate ligament, which is stronger, are less common and are sometimes seen in dashboard injuries. Treatment is surgical.

Meniscal cysts

Etiology
Meniscal cysts are similar to ganglia and develop from the lateral joint line. They may either arise from a previous joint injury or occur spontaneously. The swelling is usually most painful at night.

Management
Meniscal cysts are treated by excision.

Osteochondritis dissecans
Osteochondritis dissecans is local ischemic necrosis of bone and articular cartilage. It affects the knee more than any other joint. Osteochondral fragmentation produces loose bodies in the joint

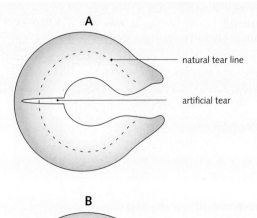

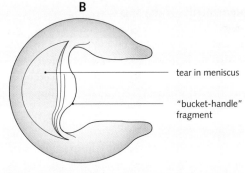

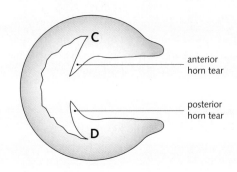

Fig. 5.19 Pattern of meniscal tears. A. The natural tear line. B. "Bucket-handle" tear (the most common type). C. Anterior horn tear. D. Posterior horn tear.

capsule. Other causes of loose bodies in the knee include OA, fracture of the joint surface, and synovial chondromatosis.

Recurrent dislocation of the patella

Etiology
The patella has a tendency to be displaced laterally every time the knee is extended, due to the valgus angle of the knee and the force vectors created by the pull of the quadriceps and patellar ligament. Predisposing factors for recurrent dislocation of the

patella include generalized ligament laxity, anatomical abnormalities of the patella or lateral condyle of the femur, or a genu valgum deformity. Recurrent dislocation of the patella tends to affect adolescent girls and often occurs bilaterally.

Clinical features
Recurrent dislocation of the patella causes severe pain in the front of the knee so that the patient cannot extend the joint and may collapse. Repeated dislocations can predispose the patient to the development of OA.

Management
Recurrent dislocation of the patella is treated by strengthening the quadriceps muscle (especially the vastus medialis muscle). If this fails, the joint needs to be stabilized surgically.

Chondromalacia patellae
Etiology
Softening of the patellar articular cartilage, or chondromalacia patellae, is an important cause of anterior knee pain, especially in teenage girls. Pain is worse when climbing up and down stairs, and there may be joint effusion.

Management
Chondromalacia patellae is treated with analgesics and by strengthening the vastus medialis muscle; surgical correction is often unsuccessful.

Osteoarthritis of the knee
Etiology
The knee is affected by OA more than other joints, especially in overweight patients with a long-standing genu varum deformity.

Clinical features
Characteristic features of OA of the knee include articular cartilage breakdown, subchondral bone sclerosis, and peripheral osteophyte formation. The patient experiences joint pain and swelling with use, leading to knee locking. The quadriceps muscle is usually wasted.

Management
Treatment of OA of the knee depends on the severity of the disease. It may be treated conservatively with analgesics and physical therapy or surgically by debridement, osteotomy, or joint replacement.

Bursitis of the knee
Bursae can become inflamed because of infection, trauma, or repeated irritating friction, giving rise to swelling and effusion. The prepatellar bursa ("housemaid's knee"), infrapatellar bursa ("vicar's knee"), and semimembranosus bursa (popliteal cyst) are commonly affected.

 A Baker's cyst is a herniation of the joint synovium backward and downward; it is not the same as a popliteal cyst.

Disorders of the ankle and foot
Congenital club foot (talipes equinovarus)
Pathology
Congenital club foot presents as inversion, marked adduction, and plantarflexion of the foot (Fig. 5.20). The calf and peroneal muscles are also underdeveloped.

Boys are affected by congenital club foot more than girls. The condition may be associated with spina bifida.

Management
Congenital club foot is corrected by splinting and/or surgery.

Pes planus and pes cavus
Pes planus (flat foot) is a flattened longitudinal arch causing the medial border of the foot to almost

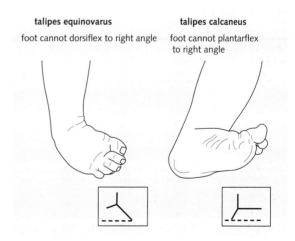

talipes equinovarus
foot cannot dorsiflex to right angle

talipes calcaneus
foot cannot plantarflex to right angle

Fig. 5.20 Features of talipes equinovarus and talipes calcaneus.

touch the ground (Fig. 5.21). It can be caused by underlying general joint laxity or can be congenital. Often there are no symptoms, but there may be foot strain and OA of the tarsal joints in later life.

Pes cavus (hollow foot) is a high longitudinal arch and may be congenital or associated with neurologic disorders, leading to weak intrinsic muscles (see Fig. 5.21). The toes may be clawed, and the metatarsal heads are prominent because they are weight-bearing.

Hammer toe

In hammer toe, the toe is flexed at the PIP joint and extended at the MTP joint (Fig. 5.22). The second toes are most commonly affected. The disorder is treated by lengthening the tendons and excising the MTP joint capsule to straighten the deformity (see Fig. 5.22).

Claw toe

In claw toe, the toe is flexed at both the PIP and DIP joints, and it is extended at the MTP joint (see Fig. 5.22). Claw toe occurs in rheumatoid arthritis and after poliomyelitis and are treated by a flexor-extensor transfer operation.

Mallet toe

In patients with mallet toe (a variant of hammer toe), there is damage to the extensor tendon (also most commonly of the second toe) at its insertion into the distal phalanx, causing a fixed flexion deformity. The DIP joint cannot be extended fully. Mallet toe is treated by placing a splint onto each toe, with the DIP joint fully extended. Before skeletal maturity, a simple flexor tenotomy will relieve the deformity.

Hallux valgus

In patients with hallux valgus (Fig. 5.23), the big toe deviates laterally at the MTP joint, and a protective bursa (bunion) develops where the shoe rubs. This condition may lead to hammer toes, bursitis, metatarsalgia, and secondary OA of the MTP joint. The wearing of high heels with pointed toes may contribute to this deformity; the condition is seen in older adult women.

Hallux rigidus
Etiology

Joint stiffness in the big toe, or hallux rigidus, may be due to OA of the MTP joint, trauma, gout, or osteochondritis dissecans in the head of the first metatarsal bone. The patient experiences pain when walking and limited movement.

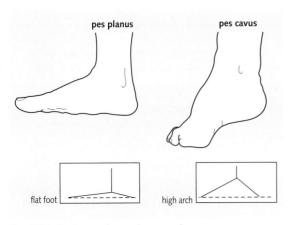

Fig. 5.21 Features of pes planus and pes cavus.

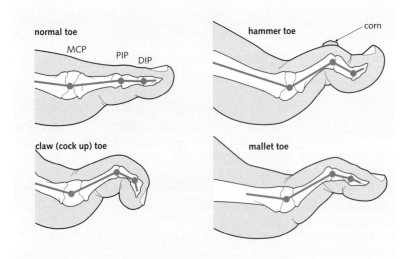

Fig. 5.22 Toe deformities: normal toe, claw (cock up) toe, hammer toe, and mallet toe.

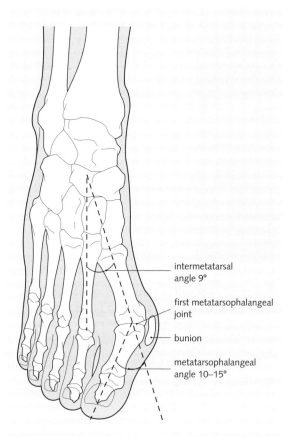

Fig. 5.23 Hallux valgus.

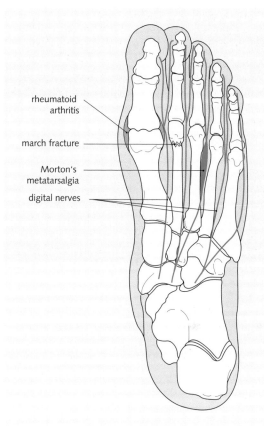

Fig. 5.24 Causes of forefoot pain.

Epidemiology

Men are more commonly affected with hallux rigidus than women.

Management

Treatment of hallux rigidus involves dealing with the underlying cause, then replacing the joint if necessary.

Forefoot pain (metatarsalgia)

Forefoot pain may be caused by foot or toe deformities (e.g., pes planus, pes cavus, hallux valgus, claw toes); it also occurs in stress fractures and Morton's metatarsalgia (Fig. 5.24).

Stress fractures (march fractures)

Stress fractures occur in the shaft of the second or third metatarsals of young adults after excessive walking. The fractures are treated by resting and wearing a plaster cast during healing.

Morton's metatarsalgia (plantar digital neuritis)

Morton's metatarsalgia is a fibrous thickening of a digital nerve between the metatarsals. Tight or ill-fitting shoes cause compressional pain in this region, which then radiates to the third and fourth toes. Wearing rubber pads or excising the thickened nerve segment alleviates the pain.

Rheumatoid arthritis in the ankle and foot

Rheumatoid arthritis affects the ankle and foot joints similar to how the arthritis affects the wrist and hands; however, in this case, there is the added complication of applying pressure on these joints when walking. The patient also experiences subluxation of the metatarsal heads, with hallux valgus, clawed toes, and prominent calluses that cause pain.

Toenail lesions
Ingrown toenails

Ingrown toenails are nails that have become embedded in the lateral skin folds and have formed

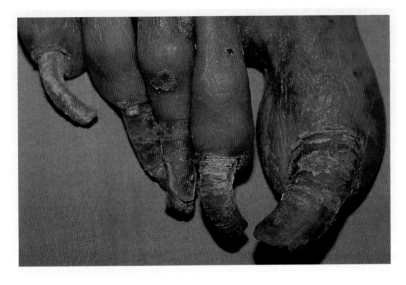

Fig. 5.25 Overgrown toenails (courtesy of Dr. G White and the Department of Dermatology, UCSD).

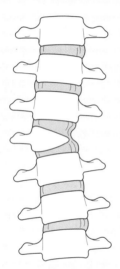

Fig. 5.26 Hemivertebrae in the spine, producing scoliosis.

inflamed (sometimes pus-filled) ulcerations. Ingrown toenails can be prevented by the correct cutting of the nails and are treated by inserting gauze under the ingrown edges of the nail to separate them from the skin fold or by removal of a sliver of the ingrown portion of the nail and its germinal matrix.

Overgrown toenails (onychogryphosis)
Overgrown toenails are very thick, hard, and curved laterally (Fig. 5.25). They are treated by excision.

Undergrown toenails (subungual exostosis)
Undergrown toenails have a bony outgrowth (exostosis) from the dorsal surface of the distal phalanx that pushes the nail upwards. They are treated by excision of the exostosis.

Disorders of the back
Congenital abnormalities
Lumbarization and sacralization are inconsequential anatomical anomalies. Lumbarization is a condition in which S1 remains as a vertebra, and sacralization refers to fusion of the body of L5 with the sacrum. Hemivertebrae are congenital abnormalities characterized by vertebrae being formed on one lateral side only (Fig. 5.26). The vertebral body is therefore wedge-shaped, causing the spine to angle laterally at this site.

Torticollis
Torticollis is a contracted sternocleidomastoid muscle on one side of the neck only. The most common cause is neck trauma during delivery. The head is tilted and rotated to one side, and there is facial asymmetry (Fig. 5.27). Torticollis is corrected by surgery.

Scoliosis
Scoliosis is the lateral curvature of the spine (Fig. 5.28). The deformity may be mobile (reversible) or fixed (permanent). Mobile scoliosis may be postural, compensatory (to a short leg or pelvic tilt), or sciatic (with disc prolapse and muscle spasm).

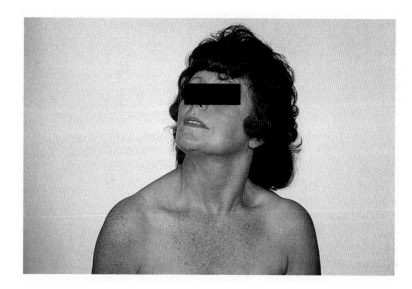

Fig. 5.27 Features of torticollis (courtesy of Dr GD Perkin).

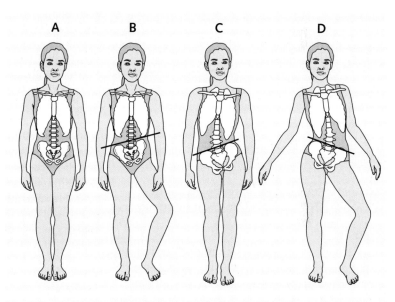

Fig. 5.28 Types of scoliosis. A. Normal posture. B. Scoliosis due to sciatica. C. Short leg. D. Fixed deformity.

Etiology

Fixed scoliosis can be caused by:

- Congenital vertebral abnormalities.
- Hemivertebrae.
- Asymmetrical muscle weakness.
- Muscular dystrophies.

Fixed scoliosis may be idiopathic in infants and adolescents.

Management

Fixed scoliosis can be treated either conservatively (with exercise or by wearing supportive splints) or surgically.

Kyphosis

Kyphosis is excessive posterior curvature of the spine that is either gently rounded or sharply angled (Fig. 5.29). It can be a progressive deformity. Kyphosis can

113

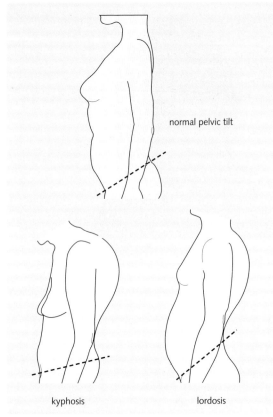

Fig. 5.29 Features of kyphosis and lordosis: normal posture, kyphosis, and lordosis.

be caused by tuberculosis of the spine, fractured vertebrae, ankylosing spondylitis, and spinal tumors.

Lordosis

Lordosis is excessive anterior curvature of the spine, usually in the lumbar region (see Fig. 5.29). It may be caused by bad posture or be compensatory for hip deformities. Lordosis may cause chronic low back pain.

Disc prolapse

Disc prolapse usually occurs in the lumbar region— the nucleus pulposus herniates through a weak part of the annulus fibrosus (Fig. 5.30). Sudden pain can be felt in the lumbar region (lumbago) or, if there is compression of a nerve root, it may radiate to the buttocks and legs (sciatica). The patient experiences limitation in flexion and extension of the lower limbs.

Management

Disc prolapse can be treated with analgesics, by injection of chymopapain (dissolves the protruding disc), or surgically, by disc excision.

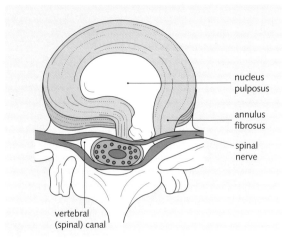

Fig. 5.30 Intervertebral disc prolapse.

Spondylolisthesis

In patients with spondylolisthesis, there is forward displacement of a lumbar vertebral body onto the one below. There may be pain, and a "step" can be palpated over the spine.

The condition can be treated conservatively by wearing a corset or surgically by fusion of the vertebral joints.

Vertebral (spinal) stenosis

Vertebral or spinal stenosis is narrowing of the vertebral (spinal) canal. It may be caused by long-term OA and disc degeneration. Standing and walking lead to severe pain in the buttocks and thighs because nerves and blood vessels are cramped. The pain is relieved by rest. Vertebral stenosis is treated by the removal of osteophytes and part of the bony canal.

Back strain

Without an adequate warm-up, the muscles and ligaments of the lumbar spine can be strained during unaccustomed or sudden movements. Back strain is treated by rest, analgesics, application of heat, and gradual mobilization.

Tuberculosis of the spine (Pott's disease)

Tuberculosis (TB) of the spine is called Pott's disease (Fig. 5.31). The spine is the most likely part of the skeleton to be affected by TB.

In patients with Pott's disease, the vertebral bodies collapse onto each other, creating a sharply angled "gibbus" deformity. There are also risks of cord compression (Pott's paraplegia), chronic discharging sinus, and the spread of TB to other organs.

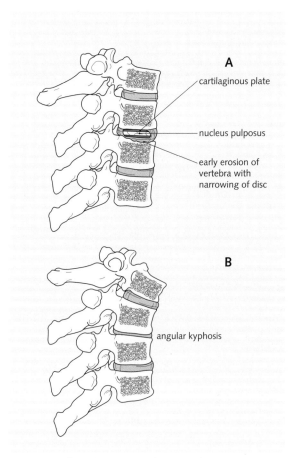

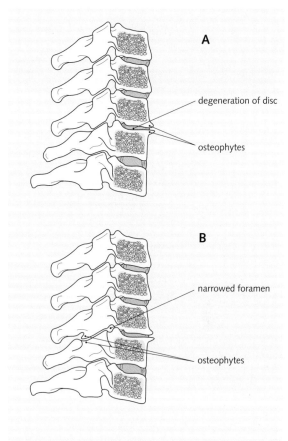

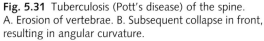

Fig. 5.31 Tuberculosis (Pott's disease) of the spine. A. Erosion of vertebrae. B. Subsequent collapse in front, resulting in angular curvature.

Fig. 5.32 Osteoarthritis of the spine. A. Degeneration and narrowing of intervertebral disc, forming osteophytes anteriorly. B. Articular cartilage that is worn away and marginal osteophytes that surround the intervertebral foramen.

Pott's disease is treated with antituberculous drugs. The pus is drained, any dead bone is removed, and the vertebrae are fused (arthrodesis).

Arthritic disease in the spine
Osteoarthritis
OA in the spine tends to affect the thoracic or lumbar vertebrae (Fig. 5.32). It usually occurs in people who lift heavy objects or those with previous injuries, such as disc prolapse or degeneration. Narrowing of the intervertebral discs and osteophyte formation in the lateral joint margins occur; these conditions predispose the patient to spinal stenosis and spondylolisthesis.

Rheumatoid arthritis
When rheumatoid arthritis occurs in the back, it often affects the cervical vertebrae. The patient experiences diffuse pain and impaired movement.

Ankylosing spondylitis
Ankylosing spondylitis affects the vertebral and sacroiliac joints before progressing to the limb joints. It occurs mostly in men. There is erosion of the normal articular cartilage and underlying bone, and then replacement with fibrous tissue occurs, and the tissue also ossifies. Derangement of the normal structures ensues. Diffuse pain, a stiffened spine, and marked restriction of chest expansion are the principal features of ankylosing spondylitis.

Pain referred to the back
Retroperitoneal disease in the abdomen (duodenal ulcer, pancreatic cancer, aortic aneurysm) may cause back pain. Period pain, labor pain, and sciatic pain also radiate to the back.

115

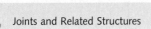
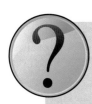

- Give a simple classification of all joints.
- Describe the different types of joints with examples.
- Describe the structure and function of synovial joints.
- Describe the blood and nerve supply and lymph drainage of joints.
- Give a simple classification of the arthropathies.
- Differentiate between the crystals found in gout and pseudogout.
- Describe the etiology of de Quervain's tenosynovitis.
- Differentiate between tennis elbow and golfer's elbow.
- List the nerve roots that refer pain to the shoulder.
- Differentiate between osteoarthritis and rheumatoid arthritis.
- Explain the difference between the pathology for vertebral (spinal) stenosis and the pathology for intermittent claudication.
- Describe the four different types of abnormal gait.
- Identify which bursae of the knee can be affected by bursitis, and name these lesions.
- Differentiate between pes cavus and pes planus.
- Name the lesions that cause the appearance of the "bamboo spine," and describe how they are formed.

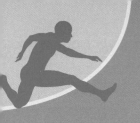

6. The Functioning Musculoskeletal System

Motor function and control

Central control of movement
Motor control
Motor systems responsible for movement have three levels of control that are organized both hierarchically and in parallel (Fig. 6.1). These levels of control are as follows:
- The cerebral cortex.
- The brainstem.
- The spinal cord.

Cerebral cortex
Three areas of the cerebral cortex are involved in motor control: the primary motor area, premotor area, and supplementary motor area. The premotor and supplementary motor areas are involved mainly in planning the sequence and strategy of complex movements, while the primary motor area is responsible for the execution of motor commands. The corticospinal tract (also known as the pyramidal tract) originates from these areas as well as from the primary somatic sensory area and is the main descending tract involved in conveying these commands to the spinal cord, which results in voluntary movement (Fig. 6.2).

Brainstem
The brainstem is the origin of other descending pathways, the so-called extrapyramidal tracts. These are the vestibulospinal, reticulospinal, and tectospinal pathways. They play a role in posture, balance, and hand-eye coordination, and they act as back-up systems when the corticospinal tract is attempting to recover following a stroke.

Spinal cord
Spinal interneurons converge on anterior horn spinal motor neurons, which innervate skeletal muscle. These interneurons act to inhibit certain muscle groups while activating others. In addition, movement can be modified by the basal ganglia and cerebellum.

Corticospinal tracts (pyramidal tracts)
The corticospinal tracts link the cerebral cortex, brainstem, and spinal cord. They originate mostly from the pyramidal neurons (giant cells of Betz) in the motor and sensory cortices, descend into the brainstem (where 80–85% of fibers cross to the opposite side), and then terminate in the gray matter of the anterior horn of the spinal cord. Lesions of the corticospinal tracts lead to upper motor neuron spastic paralysis with hyperflexia.

Coordination of movement
The coordination of movement involves, among other structures, the cerebellum and basal ganglia.

Cerebellum
The cerebellum improves the accuracy of movement by comparing actual movement (via feedback from

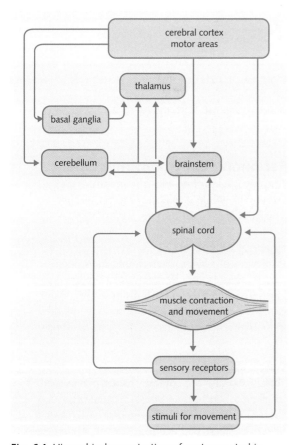

Fig. 6.1 Hierarchical organization of motor control in movement.

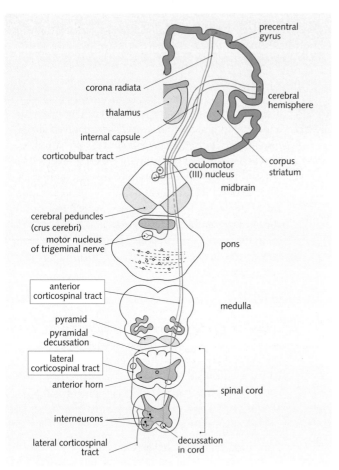

Fig. 6.2 Corticospinal tract.

the spinal cord) with intended movement (via input from the motor cortex), thus acting as a comparator. This information is passed forward to the brainstem so that movement is modified as it occurs. Cerebellar disease generally manifests as loss of balance and equilibrium accompanied by an intention tremor. These signs are known collectively as cerebellar ataxia.

Basal ganglia

Basal ganglia play an important role in the planning and coordination of movement and posture. They have connections with the thalamus and cerebral cortex and are involved in facilitating some movements while suppressing other, unwanted movements. Degeneration of neurons within the basal ganglia manifests in diseases such as Parkinson's and Huntington's, diseases in which movement disorders such as temors and dyskinesia are the hallmark.

Peripheral control of movement

Peripheral control enables the monitoring of movement, while it is occurring, via sensory receptors in skeletal muscle.

Types of receptors

Two types of receptors are found in skeletal muscle: muscle spindles and Golgi tendon organs. They are important in both proprioception and spinal reflexes. The reflexes of muscle spindles and Golgi tendon organs exert opposite effects (Fig. 6.3).

Muscle spindles

Muscle spindles are spindle-shaped organs made up of modified muscle fibers, termed intrafusal fibers (Fig. 6.4). Intrafusal fibers are narrower than extrafusal fibers and act as miniature strain gauges, continuously monitoring muscle tension (tone) as the muscle shortens during contraction.

118

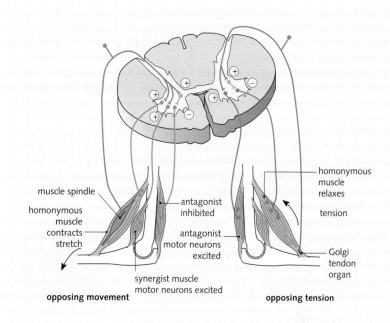

Fig. 6.3 Opposite effects of muscle spindle and Golgi tendon organ reflexes.

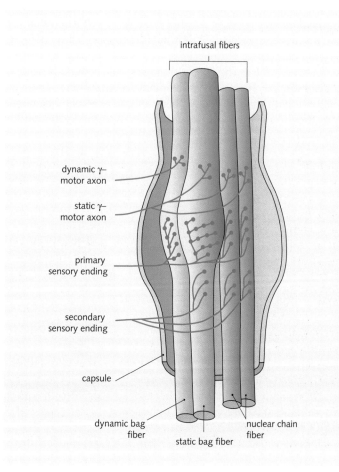

Fig. 6.4 Muscle spindle.

Because muscle spindles lie parallel to muscle fibers, they respond to changes in length. Each spindle consists of several intrafusal fibers. These include:

- Two nuclear bag fibers, one for dynamic responses and the other for static responses.
- Five to six nuclear chain fibers for static responses.

Sensory innervation of muscle spindles is performed by group Ia afferent fibers, which supply both nuclear bag and nuclear chain fibers via primary endings. Group Ia afferent fibers show static and dynamic sensitivity (i.e., they respond to stretch and its rate).

One or more group II afferent fibers form secondary endings on nuclear chain fibers, although there may be occasional contact with a nuclear bag fiber. These fibers show static sensitivity only (i.e., they respond to change in muscle length). Motor innervation of muscle spindles is important because it determines the sensitivity of muscle spindles to stretch (Fig. 6.5).

When the extrafusal fibers of muscle contract, the muscle spindle may no longer respond because its fibers are not being stretched. Activation of the γ-neurons causes shortening of the muscle spindles at the same time as the extrafusal fibers. During normal muscle contraction, descending pathways activate both the fast-conducting α-motor neurons (i.e., they stimulate extrafusal muscle contraction) and the slower-conducting γ-motor neurons (i.e., they stimulate muscle spindle contraction) at the same time. This is known as α–γ coactivation.

Dynamic γ-motor axons supply the nuclear bag fibers. When activated, they enhance the dynamic response of group Ia fibers. Static γ-motor axons supply the nuclear chain fibers. When activated, they enhance the static responses of both group Ia and II fibers. Different descending pathways preferentially activate either dynamic or static motor neurons.

Slow-conducting γ-motor axons supply intrafusal muscle fibers, while fast-conducting α-motor axons supply extrafusal, or "regular," muscle fibers.

Golgi tendon organs

Golgi tendon organs consist of the terminals of a group Ib afferent fiber. These terminals are wrapped around bundles of collagen fibers in the tendon of a muscle. These lie in series with the extrafusal fibers, responding to changes in force. There is no efferent innervation of Golgi tendon organs.

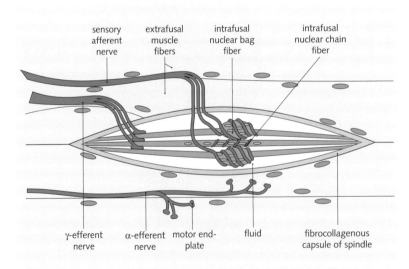

Fig. 6.5 Innervation of the muscle spindle.

Posture and locomotion

Posture
Control of posture
Posture is the relative position of the trunk, head, and limbs in space. To keep posture stable, the body's center of gravity needs to be maintained in position over its support base.

Postural reflexes correct changes in posture caused by displacement of the center of gravity—by either external forces or deliberate movement. Postural change is detected by musculoskeletal proprioceptors, the vestibular system, and the visual system.

Vestibular system
The vestibular system detects changes in head position, linear acceleration, and angular acceleration. The vestibular nuclei use this information, together with afferent nerves from the neck muscles and cervical vertebrae, to determine if the head is moving alone or if the head and the body are both moving. The nuclei can influence antigravity and axial musculature via a direct projection into the spinal cord (vestibulospinal projection).

Locomotion
Control of locomotion
Locomotion requires coordination between the systems controlling posture and those producing voluntary movement. This ensures that the body is supported against gravity and that the center of gravity lies over the support base during propulsion.

A rhythm of muscle activity is needed, because each limb takes its turn in supporting the body and moving it forward. The circuits that generate this pattern of activity are in the spinal cord and can be activated by higher centers (e.g., the brainstem). Sensory input is important in maintaining coordination of locomotion.

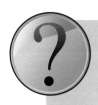

- Describe the hierarchical organization of the motor system.
- Locate the corticospinal tract (pyramidal tract) and describe its course through the brain and spinal cord.
- Describe the role of the cerebellum and the basal ganglia in coordination of movement.
- Describe the structure and innervation of muscle spindles.
- Describe the role of the central pattern generator in movement.

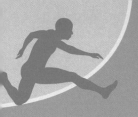

7. The Skin

Organization of the skin

The skin is the largest organ in the body, making up 16% of the body's weight, and has a surface area of 1.8 m². It has an essential role in both homeostasis and protection of the body from external influences. The skin is composed of three layers:

- The epidermis—stratified squamous epithelium.
- The dermis—supportive connective tissue matrix.
- The subcutaneous layer—loose connective tissue and fat.

The epidermis (ectoderm) develops by the first month of gestation. The dermis (mesoderm) develops at a later stage, usually at around 11 weeks. By gestational week 17, the skin ridges responsible for fingerprints have developed. The composition of the three separate layers of the skin (see Fig. 1.2) is described in the sections that follow.

Epidermis

The epidermis is generally around 0.1 mm thick, although it reaches depths of between 0.8 and 1.4 mm on the palms of the hand and soles of the feet. It is designed to withstand wear and tear, and it is made up of stratified squamous keratinized epithelium. The epidermis itself comprises four separate layers: the stratum basale (basal cell layer), the stratum spinosum (prickle cell layer), the stratum granulosum (granular cell layer), and the stratum corneum (horny layer). These four layers are formed by the differing stages of maturation of keratin (Fig. 7.1), a protein produced by keratinocytes, the main cell of the epidermis.

Stratum basale

This layer is composed of keratinocytes (90%) that may be dividing or nondividing, melanocytes (5–10%), and infrequent Merkel cells. Keratinocytes are anchored to the basement membrane by hemidesmosomes, which are essentially condensations of tonofibrils, which in turn are formed by synthesized keratin.

   Melanocytes synthesize melanins that absorb the energy of ultraviolet radiation and act as free radical scavengers. The cells originate from the neural crest and are most numerous on sites exposed to the sun. Merkel cells appear to have a role in sensation and are found close to the terminal filament of cutaneous nerves.

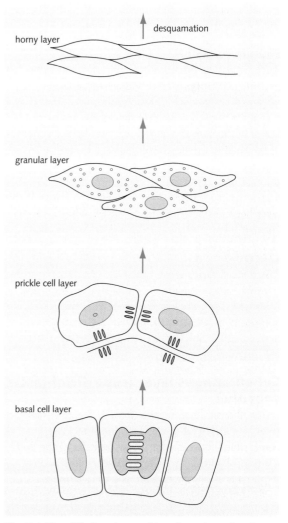

Fig. 7.1 The differing stages of keratinocyte maturation (adapted from *Dermatology: An Illustrated Colour Text*, 2nd ed., by Gawkrodger DJ, Churchill Livingstone, 1997).

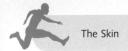

Stratum spinosum

Here, the keratinocytes change from columnar to polyhedral. Desmosomes, again made of tonofibrils, connect the cells and help distribute stress equally throughout the epidermis as well as help maintain a distance of 20 nm between adjacent cells. When seen under a light microscope, these desmosomes form the "prickles" that give the layer its name. Langerhans cells are also found in this layer; these are dendritic cells derived from the bone marrow and play an important role in the cellular immune system.

Stratum granulosum

As the keratinocytes mature, the cells flatten and lose their nuclei. The cytoplasm gains keratohyalin granules and membrane-coating granules that burst their contents into the intercellular spaces.

Stratum corneum

At the end of the maturation process, the keratocytes become overlapping, cornified cells that lack a nucleus—corneocytes. The cytoplasm is replaced by a matrix composed of keratin tonofibrils and keratohyalin granules, glued together by the contents of the membrane-coating granules. This horny layer forms the outermost layer of the skin. The keratin provides flexibility and strength, and the corneocyte layer can absorb three times its weight in water. If the layer becomes dehydrated, however, with the water content falling to below 10%, it is no longer pliable.

Dermis

The dermis varies greatly in thickness, ranging from 0.6 mm on the eyelids to 3 mm on the palms and soles. It is found below the epidermis and is composed of a tough, supportive cell matrix containing fibroblasts, dermal dendrocytes, mast cells, lymphocytes, and macrophages.

Subcutaneous layer (superficial fascia subcutis)

Situated directly under the dermis, the subcutaneous layer or superficial fascia is made up of loose connective tissue and fat. Most fat cells in the body are housed in this layer, and these subcutaneous fat deposits are collectively referred to as adipose tissue.

Skin physiology

Keratinocytes, the basic building blocks of the skin, take around 14 days to mature fully as they travel from the basal layer to the stratum corneum; the dividing cells in the stratum basale replicate every 200–400 hours. In another 14 days, the dead corneocytes are shed from the horny layer of the skin in a process called desquamation. This cell turnover rate of 28 days is dramatically shortened in keratinization disorders such as psoriasis.

Keratinocytes are also involved in the pathology of the blistering skin disorders. Circulating IgG autoantibodies, which are detectable in the serum by indirect immunofluorescence in 90% of affected patients, bind to components in the intercellular epidermal substance and induce proteolytic enzyme release from the adjacent keratinocytes. These enzymes cause the loss of adhesion between cells and result in splits in the epidermis.

Derivative structures of the skin

Hair

Humans no longer rely on hair to play a vital role in the conservation of heat—humans are relatively hairless compared to most other mammals. Although scalp hair still protects against the harmful effects of ultraviolet radiation and minor injuries, the main roles of hair today are of appearance and sexual attraction.

Hair can be found in varying densities of growth over the entire surface of the body; exceptions are the vulval introitus, glans penis, and the glabrous skin of the palms and soles of the feet. Follicles are most dense on the scalp and face. Follicles are derived from the epidermis (cells of the cortex matrix and the hair shaft) and the dermis (papilla).

Structure of hair

Each hair follicle is lined by germinative cells that produce keratin and the other components of the hair shaft. The hair shaft itself consists of an outer cuticle, a cortex of keratinocytes, and an inner medulla (Fig.7.2). The root sheath that surrounds the hair bulb is composed of an inner and outer layer. An arrector pili muscle is associated with the hair shaft, which is the structure behind "goose bumps"—it contracts with cold, fear, and emotion to pull the hair erect.

Classification of hair types

There are three types of hair:
- Lanugo hairs—These are formed at gestational week 20 and are usually shed before the fetus is

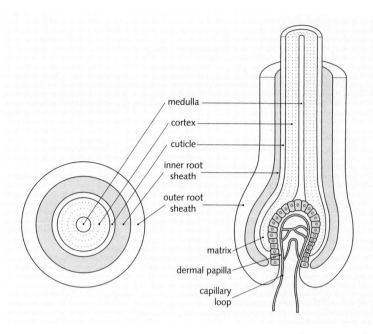

Fig 7.2 Structure of hair follicle (adapted from *Dermatology: An Illustrated Colour Text,* 2nd ed., by Gawkrodger DJ, Churchill Livingstone, 1997).

born. They can be seen in premature babies and are fine and long.

- Vellus hairs—This is the most common hair type; vellus hairs cover most of the surface of the body. They are short, fine, and light in color.
- Terminal hairs—There are around 100,000 terminal hairs on the scalp, and they are also found in the eyebrows, eyelashes, and the pubic and axillary regions. They are also the hairs that compose the beard.

Stages of hair development

Hair growth is cyclical, with the normal rate being 0.4 mm per day. There are three different stages of hair development (Fig. 7.3) as the following describes.

Anagen: This is the growth phase; between 80% and 90% of scalp hair is in this phase at any one time. The length of this phase depends on the hair site: it lasts between 3 and 7 years for scalp hair but only 4 months for eyebrow hair.

Catagen: The resting phase normally lasts for 3–4 weeks. During this stage, the synthesis of the hair follicle stops. Between 10% and 20% of scalp hair is in catagen at any one time, with 50–100 follicles entering the phase every day.

Telogen: This is the shedding phase; less than 1% of scalp hairs are in telogen at any one time. Hairs

undergoing telogen are distinguished by a short club root.

Hair growth is not usually in phase, but if it is synchronized during the resting stage, it will be uniformly shed 3 months later (telogen effluvium). This synchronization results from childbirth, high fever, surgery, drugs, or other stress. Anagen effluvium (abrupt cessation of hair growth) occurs after ingestion of drugs such as cytotoxins, heparin and warfarin, carbimazole, colchicine, and vitamin A. It may also follow ingestion of drugs such as thallium.

Nails

Consisting of a dense plate of hardened keratin between 0.3 mm and 0.5 mm thick, the nail is a leftover of the mammalian claw. Its function is to protect the tip of the finger, increase the tactile sensitivity of the pulp of the finger, and facilitate grasping.

Structure of the nail

The nail is composed of a nail bed, nail matrix, and a nail plate (Fig. 7.4). The nail matrix (nail bed underneath the base or root of the nail plate) is composed of dividing keratinocytes that mature and keratinize into the nail plate. The nail bed lies underneath the main body of the nail plate; this bed produces a small amount of keratin. The pink appearance of the nail plate is caused by the dermal

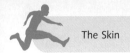

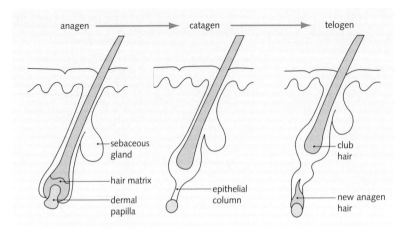

Fig. 7.3 Stage of hair development (adapted from *Dermatology: An Illustrated Colour Text*, 2nd ed., by Gawkrodger DJ, Churchill Livingstone, 1997).

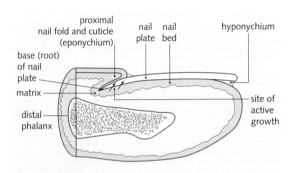

Fig. 7.4 Structure of the nail (adapted from *Dermatology: An Illustrated Colour Text*, 2nd ed., by Gawkrodger DJ, Churchill Livingstone, 1997).

capillaries that underlie the nail, and the white lunula at the base of the nail plate is the distal, visible part of the nail matrix. The thickened epidermis that underlies the free margin of the nail at the proximal end is called the hyponychium.

Nail growth

The fingernails grow at the rate of 0.1 mm per day; the toenails grow more slowly. Any pathologic process that disturbs nail growth leaves visible clinical signs in the nail. Systemic illness may lead to transverse grooves in the nail called Beau's lines, which indicate an interruption to the growth of the nail matrix. Cytotoxic drugs cause black transverse bands in the nail, heavy metal poisoning causes white transverse bands, and trauma to the nail matrix can cause white spots within the nail or splinter hemorrhages.

Clubbing of the nail is caused by many disorders (Fig. 7.5); the nail matrix increases in vascularity and

feels fluctuant. In addition, the normal angle between the base of the nail and the nail fold is lost, the nail curvature increases in all directions, and the end of the finger may expand.

Sebaceous glands

Derived from epidermal cells, sebaceous glands are closely associated with hair follicles and produce an oily sebum (Fig. 7.6). This sebum flows into the hair follicles; from there, sebum travels to the surface of the skin, where it oils both the hair and the keratinized surface of the skin to help waterproof and protect them from dehydrating and cracking. The secretions are in general highly toxic to bacteria.

The sebaceous glands are sensitive to androgens and become active at puberty. They are most numerous over the scalp, face, chest, and back and are not present on hairless skin.

Sweat glands

Sweat glands are located in the dermis and are present over the majority of the body—there are an estimated 2.5 million on the skin's surface. The glands are composed of coiled tubes that secrete a watery substance and are classified into two different types: eccrine and apocrine.

Eccrine glands

Eccrine glands are sweat glands found all over the skin, especially in the palms, soles, axillae, and forehead; they are not present in mucous membranes. Eccrine glands are under psychological and thermal control and are innervated by sympathetic (cholinergic) nerve fibers. The watery

Causes of finger clubbing	
Respiratory	Lung cancer, cystic fibrosis, interstitial lung disease, idiopathic pulmonary fibrosis, sarcoidosis, lipoid pneumonia, empyema, pleural mesothelioma, pulmonary artery sarcoma, cryptogenic fibrosing alveolitis, pulmonary metastases, bronchiectasis, and lung abscess
Cardiac	Cyanotic congenital heart disease, other causes of right-to-left shunting, and bacterial endocarditis
Gastrointestinal	Ulcerative colitis, Crohn's disease, primary biliary cirrhosis, cirrhosis of the liver, achalasia, and peptic ulceration of the esophagus
Malignancy	Thyroid cancer, thymus cancer, Hodgkin's disease, and disseminated chronic myeloid leukemia
Miscellaneous	Acromegaly, thyroid acropachy, and pregnancy

Fig. 7.5 Some causes of finger clubbing (adapted from *Principles of Clinical Medicine*, 2nd ed., Kumar PJ and Clarke ML, Bailliere Tindall, 1990).

Location of sebaceous sweat glands	
Type of gland	**Location**
Sebaceous	Associated with hair follicles; found on scalp, face, chest, and back. They are not found on skin that is hairless.
Eccrine sweat	Widely distributed, but most numerous on palms, soles, axillae, and forehead
Apocrine sweat	Open into hair follicles; profuse around axillae, perineum, and areolae

Fig. 7.6 Location of sebaceous and sweat glands (adapted from *Principles of Clinical Medicine*, 2nd ed., Kumar PJ and Clarke ML, Bailliere Tindall, 1990).

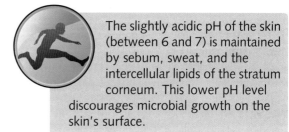 The slightly acidic pH of the skin (between 6 and 7) is maintained by sebum, sweat, and the intercellular lipids of the stratum corneum. This lower pH level discourages microbial growth on the skin's surface.

fluid that the glands secrete contains chloride, lactic acid, fatty acids, urea, glycoproteins, and mucopolysaccharides.

Apocrine glands

Apocrine glands are large sweat glands with ducts that empty out into the hair follicles. They are present in the axillae, anogenital region, and areolae. They become active at puberty and produce an odorless, protein-rich secretion that gives out a characteristic odor when acted upon by skin bacteria. The apocrine glands are a phylogenetic remnant of the mammalian sexual scent gland. Wax in the ears is produced by a modified version of the same gland. Apocrine glands are also present on the eyelids. These glands are under the control of the sympathetic (adrenergic) nerve fibers.

Nerves in the skin

Functions of the skin include perception of touch, pain, and temperature, so the organ is richly innervated. The densest concentrations of nerve endings are found in areas where sensation is of paramount importance: hands, face, and genitalia. Different types of sensation detectors are found in the skin (Fig. 7.7). Free sensory nerve endings are found in the dermis and epidermis, and they detect pain, itch, and temperature. They contain neuropeptide transmitters, such as substance P. Corpuscular receptors, which are specialized for certain types of sensation, are also found in the dermis: these are Pacinian corpuscles, which detect pressure and vibration, and Meissner's corpuscles, which are sensitive to touch. These corpuscles are found in the dermal papillae of the feet and hands. Innervation to hair-bearing and nonhair-bearing skin is also different.

Merkel cells are derived embryologically from the neural crest and play a role in sensation by acting as mechanoreceptors to pick up sustained pressure on the skin. They also contain

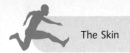

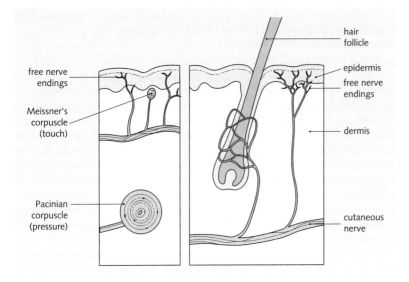

free nerve endings

Meissner's corpuscle (touch)

Pacinian corpuscle (pressure)

hair follicle

epidermis

free nerve endings

dermis

cutaneous nerve

Fig. 7.7 The different types of nerve receptors in the skin (adapted from *Dermatology: An Illustrated Colour Text,* 2nd ed., by Gawkrodger DJ, Churchill Livingstone, 1997).

neurotransmitters. The sensory nerve fibers that innervate the skin are both myelinated and unmyelinated, and their cell bodies are contained within the dorsal root ganglia of the spinal nerves.

Vessels in the skin

The skin has a rich blood supply. A superficial arterial plexus is formed at the papillary and reticular dermal boundary by branches of the subcutis artery. Branches from this plexus form capillary loops in the papillae of the dermis, each with a singular arterial and venous vessel: arteriovenous anastomoses. The veins drain into the middermal and subcutaneous venous plexus.

Dilation or contraction of the arteriovenous anastomoses plays a direct role in thermoregulation of the skin. The changes in blood flow through the capillary loops help to control direct heat loss through the surface of the skin via convection and radiation (Fig. 7.8). The arteriovenous anastomoses are under the control of the sympathetic nervous system.

Lymphatic drainage of the skin occurs through lymphatic networks that originate in the papillae and go on to become larger lymphatic vessels, which subsequently drain into regional lymph nodes.

Functions of the skin

Skin performs several functions. These include:
- Providing a mechanical barrier to antigens and bacteria, thus forming a protective cover for the body.

- Contributing to thermoregulation.
- Synthesizing vitamin D in the epidermis upon exposure to sunlight.
- Providing protection against excessive water absorption or loss.
- Providing protection against wear and tear on the surface of the body.
- Providing protection, via skin pigmentation, against ultraviolet light.
- Distinguishing between pain, touch, and temperature sensations.

Keratinocyte function

The main function of keratinocytes is to produce the high-molecular-weight polypeptide chains called keratin. The stages of keratinocyte maturation have been described. Each different stage of keratinocyte maturation produces different molecular weight keratins (e.g., 50, 55, 57, and 67 kDa); hence, different keratins are found in each separate layer of the epidermis. The hardness of keratin is caused by the strong covalent bonds that link the cysteine molecules, and the keratin found in the epidermis contains less cysteine and more glycine molecules than the stronger keratin that makes up hair.

Melanocyte function

Melanocytes are found in the basal layer of the epidermis and produce melanin, a brownish pigment that protects against harmful ultraviolet rays from the sun—the melanin forms a protective cap over the nuclei of keratinocytes in the epidermis. The

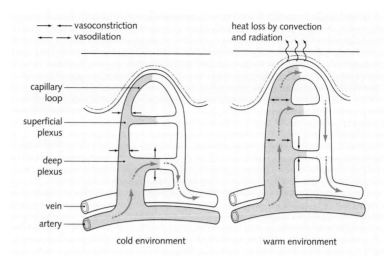

Fig. 7.8 Regulation of temperature by arteriovenous anastomoses (adapted from *Dermatology: An Illustrated Colour Text,* 2nd ed., by Gawkrodger DJ, Churchill Livingstone, 1997).

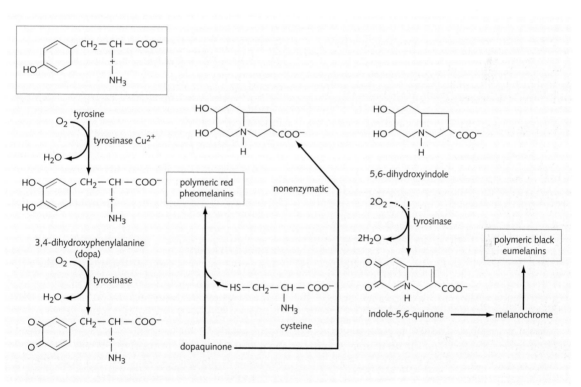

Fig. 7.9 Biosynthesis of melanin from tyrosine (adapted from *Dermatology: An Illustrated Colour Text,* 2nd ed., by Gawkrodger DJ, Churchill Livingstone, 1997).

hereditary determination of the number and size of melanosomes, the membrane-bound storage organelles, is responsible for the varying shades of the skin across different races and not the number of melanocytes. In addition, the amount of melanin in the skin can be temporarily increased in response to exposure to the sun's rays, because preformed melanin is photo-oxidized, stimulating melanocytes to produce more melanin. The result is a "tan."

In addition to absorbing the energy of ultraviolet radiation, melanin also acts as a free radical scavenger and as an energy sink. Melanin itself is produced from tyrosine (Fig. 7.9) and comes in two separate forms, eumelanin and pheomelanin. Eumelanin is the more common form and pigments the skin a brown-black color. Pheomelanin produces a yellow-red coloration and is the pigment produced in red-haired people. Most melanins are a mixture of the two different forms.

Fibroblast function

Fibroblasts produce and secrete the components of the extracellular matrix, the intricate meshwork of fibrous proteins embedded in a gel-like substance. The extracellular matrix holds the cells together, so the majority of the cells are not in direct physical contact with each other. Nutrients, waste products, and other water-soluble materials diffuse through the gelatinous matrix between the blood vessels and cell tissues.

The main components of the extracellular matrix produced by fibroblasts are collagen, elastin, and structural proteoglycans, such as glycosaminoglycans (GAGs). Their functions are discussed in Chapter 1. Collagen is the major structural protein of the dermis and makes up 70–80% of its dry weight. Of the 15 different types of collagen, 5 are found in the skin (Fig. 7.10).

The cable-like structure of collagen fibers provides tensile strength; the collagen is resistant to longitudinal stress. For disorders characterized by pathology of the collagen, such as scurvy (a disease caused by vitamin C deficiency), the tissues that rely on collagen for strength become very fragile. In skin, the blood vessels are easily damaged, and bleeding is very noticeable in the mucous membranes, especially in the gums.

Elastin is a rubber band-like protein fiber that facilitates the stretching and recoiling of structures. It plays an important role in the inflation and deflation of the lungs; in the skin, elastin maintains normal elasticity and flexibility. In large arteries, such as the aorta, it facilitates the propagation of blood through pulsations of the arterial wall.

The structural proteoglycans that make up the ground substance of the skin are mainly GAGs; these proteins are responsible for the viscosity and hydration of the skin.

Thermoregulation

Thermoregulation is dependent on metabolic and physical factors. The evaporation of sweat from the skin's surface aids cooling of the skin, and the variations in the arteriovenous anastomoses also play an important role in temperature regulation. Both of these mechanisms help to maintain the body's core temperature of 37°C in differing climates and during physical exertion.

Immune functions of the skin

The skin's structures, cells, functional systems, and immunogenetics all play a role in the cutaneous immunity system (Fig 7.11).

Epidermal barrier

The epidermal barrier is a physical structure that is impenetrable to most microorganisms that come into contact with it. In addition to this external structure, the vessels of the dermis are important routes through which immune cells can travel to where they are needed.

Langerhans cells

Situated in the epidermis, the dendritic, bone marrow-derived Langerhans cells are the first line of defense against microorganisms that penetrate the epidermal barrier. They can be distinguished histologically by Birbeck's granules, a cytoplasmic organelle found only in this type of cell. The Langerhans cells play a defensive role in antigen presentation.

Type of collagen	Location
Type I	Reticular dermis
Type III	Papillary dermis
Types IV and VII	Basement membrane structures
Type VIII	Endothelial cells

Fig. 7.10 Types of collagen found in the skin.

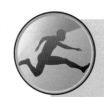

Other dendritic cells can be distinguished in the epidermis and also appear to present antigen. If they lack the Birbeck's granules, however, they are not Langerhans cells.

Immune components of the skin		
Type defense	**Different components**	**Action**
Structural	Skin	Impenetrable physical barrier to most outside organisms
	Blood and lymphatic channels	Provide transport network for cellular defense
Cellular	Langerhans cells	Play important role in antigen presentation
	T lymphocytes	Facilitate immune reactions, including cell destruction; self-regulating through the action of suppressor T cells
	Mast cells	Facilitate inflammatory reaction of the skin
	Keratinocytes	Produce inflammatory cytokines; have the ability to express surface immunoreactive molecules
Systematic	Skin-associated lymphoid tissue	Since skin contains the above immune cells and structural defenses, it can be classified as a fully functioning immunologic unit
	Cytokines and eicosanoids	Cytokines are cell mediation molecules produced by components of the cellular defense system; eicosanoids are nonspecific inflammatory mediators produced by mast cells, macrophages, and keratinocytes
	Complement cascade	Activation of the complement cascade initiates a variety of destructive mechanisms, including opsonization, lysis, chemotaxis, and mast cell degranulation
	Adhesion molecules	Increase the number of cellular defense facilitators in a particular area by binding T cells
Immunogenetic	Major histocompatibility complex (MHC)	Facilitates immunologic recognition of antigens; located on HLA gene cluster; the appearance of specific HLA genes is associated with certain pathologies (e.g., ankylosing spondylitis is associated with HLA B27)

Fig. 7.11 Immune components of the skin.

T lymphocytes

The T lymphocytes (also called T cells) are produced in the bone marrow and mature in the thymus gland; they circulate throughout the body's tissues and come into direct contact with invading foreign antigens. Once activated by this binding process, the T lymphocytes proliferate and carry out a cell-mediated immune attack on the antigens.

There are four different types of T lymphocytes (Fig. 7.12) that are distinguished by their functions and varying surface receptors and identified by monoclonal antibodies. The other family of lymphocytes, B lymphocytes, is not normally seen in the skin but can be present in some types of skin pathology.

Mast cells

Mast cells are found in the dermis and are involved in the immediate (type I) hypersensitivity reaction of the skin. They can be recruited to inflammation sites in the dermis.

Keratinocytes

As well as being responsible for keratin, keratinocytes produce proinflammatory cytokines, such as interleukin-1 (IL-1). Keratinocytes can also express surface immune reactive molecules, such as major histocompatibility complex (MHC) class II antigens (e.g., human leukocyte antigen [HLA] DR), and intercellular cell adhesion molecules (ICAM), such as ICAM-1.

MHC class II antigens are also expressed on B lymphocytes, Langerhans cells, macrophages, endothelial cells, and some T lymphocytes. They play an important role in immunologic recognition and are also responsible for the mechanism behind transplant rejection. The tissue-type antigens of each person are also found in the MHC, which is situated in the HLA

131

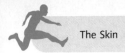

T lymphocytes found in the skin	
Helper	Facilitates immune reactions
Delayed hypersensitivity	Specifically sensitized
Cytotoxic	Kills infecting cells
Suppressor	Regulates other lymphocytes

Fig. 7.12 T lymphocytes found in the skin.

HLA antigens associated with skin diseases	
Skin disease	HLA antigen
Psoriasis	B13, Bw37, Cw23
Reiter's disease	B27
Dermatitis herpetiformis	B8

Fig. 7.13 HLA antigens associated with skin diseases.

gene complex on chromosome 6. Certain HLA genes are associated with an increased risk of developing specific diseases, including some that are classified as "autoimmune" (Fig. 7.13).

The adhesion molecules, in particular ICAM-1, are found on the cell surface of lymphocytes and some endothelial cells and keratinocytes. They bind with T cells by interacting with leukocyte-functional antigens and thus increase the site's cell traffic.

Lymphoid tissues of the skin
Lymphoid tissue is a term used to describe tissues that collectively store, produce, and process lymphocytes. The skin, with its rich blood supply and generous lymphatic drainage, together with the circulating T lymphocytes and *in situ* immune cells, can be classified as lymphoid tissue.

Cytokines and eicosanoids
The cytokines include γ-interferon, IL-1, IL-2, and IL-3. Produced mainly by T lymphocytes, these soluble molecules mediate actions between cells. They are also produced by Langerhans cells, keratinocytes, fibroblasts, endothelial cells, and macrophages.

Eicosanoids are produced from arachidonic acids by mast cells, macrophages, and keratinocytes. They are nonspecific inflammatory mediators; prostaglandins, thromboxanes, and leukotrienes are all eicosanoids.

Hypersensitivity reactions of the skin
A hypersensitivity reaction is one in which the adaptive immune response is exaggerated or inappropriate; an allergy is the acquisition of an inappropriate specific immune reaction to a normally harmless substance in the environment. There are four main types of hypersensitivity response, all of which are exhibited in the skin (Fig 7.14)

 If a patient who has high circulating levels of a certain antibody is injected with the appropriate antigen, an Arthus reaction will occur—a type III hypersensitivity reaction. This involves a red edematous area that develops over the site of the injection within 4–12 hours.

Skin secretions
The components of sweat, sebum, and epidermal lipids differ in content (Fig. 7.15). Sweat is a watery isotonic liquid that is delivered to the skin's surface. It has a low pH of between 4 and 6.8 that makes the skin slightly acidic, and this discourages microbial growth. The minimum insensible loss through perspiration per day is 0.5 L/h, and the maximum daily output is 10 L, which is limited by the body's capability of sweating 2 L/h. Men sweat more than women. In addition to lowering the skin's pH and cooling the skin, sweat hydrates the outer layers of the epidermis and aids the hands and soles of the feet in gripping.

Hormonal production and the skin
The skin manufactures vitamin D in the dermis but is also affected by many other hormones (Fig. 7.16).

Hypersensitivity reactions of the skin	
Type I (intermediate)	Fc receptors bind IgE to the surface of mast cells; when an antigen is encountered, the IgE molecules cross-link. This action stimulates the release of inflammatory mediators such as histamine, prostaglandins, and leukotrienes. The response occurs within minutes, although there is a delayed component present, which results in urticaria in the skin. Massive histamine release can cause anaphylaxis. The most common allergens that provoke an allergic reaction are pollen grains, bee stings, penicillin, certain foods, molds, and house dust mites.
Type II (antibody-dependent cytotoxicity)	When antigens bind to target skin cells on the basement membrane, a reaction occurs whereby cytotoxic killer T cells or complement activation destroy the foreign body. The powerful effects of complement cascade activation include opsonization, lysis, mast cell degranulation, smooth muscle contraction, and chemotaxis. Hemolytic anemia and transfusion reactions are examples of type II hypersensitivity, as is the pathology involved in pemphigus: IgG antibodies that are directed against keratinocyte surface-antigens result in lysis of the keratinocytes, causing intraepidermal splitting. This results in characteristic skin blisters of pemphigus.
Type III (immune complex disease)	When antigens and antibodies bind in the blood, an immune complex is formed, which is deposited in the walls of small blood vessels such as those found in the skin. Although these complexes are usually removed by the reticuloendothelial system, a leukocytoclastic vasculitis can sometimes occur; vascular damage is caused by complement activation and lysosomal enzymes released from polymorphs. This vasculitis is seen in systemic lupus erythematosus, dermatomyositis, and microbial infections such as infective endocarditis.
Type IV (cell-mediated or delayed)	Presensitized T cells come into secondary contact with the antigen after it has become bound to an antigen-presenting cell. The T cells release cytokines, which in turn activate other T cells and macrophages—the process takes some time, and the damage to tissue is most pronounced after 48–72 hours. Disorders that contain a variant of type IV hypersensitivity in their pathology include allergic contact dermatitis, leprosy, and tuberculosis.

Fig. 7.14 Hypersensitivity reactions of the skin (adapted from *Dermatology: An Illustrated Colour Text,* 2nd ed., by Gawkrodger DJ, Churchill Livingstone, 1997).

Components of sebum and epidermal lipid		
Component	Sebum (%)	Epidermal lipid (%)
Glyceride/free fatty acids	58	65
Wax esters	26	0
Squalene	12	0
Cholesterol esters	3	15
Cholesterol	1	20

Fig. 7.15 Components of sebum and epidermal lipid.

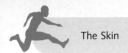

Action of hormones on the skin		
Hormone	**Site of production**	**Action on skin**
Corticosteroids	Adrenal cortex	Vasoconstriction, decreased mitosis of basal cells, anti-inflammatory role
Androgens	Adrenal cortex, gonads	Stimulates growth of terminal hair, stimulates sebum production
Estrogens	Adrenal cortex, ovaries	Stimulates melanin production
Melanocyte-stimulating hormone (MSH)	Pituitary gland	Stimulates melanin production
Adrenocorticotrophic hormone (ACTH)	Pituitary gland	Stimulates melanin production
Epidermal growth factor (EGF)	Skin	Stimulates cell differentiation, plays a role in calcium metabolism
Vitamin D	Skin	No effect on skin, plays a role in bone metabolism

Fig. 7.16 Hormones and the skin.

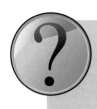

- List the four different sections of the epidermis, and describe the stage of keratinocyte maturation for each one.
- Define where you would find lanugo, vellus, and terminal hair.
- List 10 causes of clubbing.
- Differentiate between eccrine and apocrine sweat glands.
- Describe the different functions of Merkel's cells, Meissner's corpuscles, and Pacinian corpuscles.
- Describe the two forms of melanin.
- List the various products of fibroblasts and their functions.
- Describe the four different types of hypersensitivity reaction.
- List the functions of sweat.
- Explain the systemic importance of vitamin D production.

8. Disorders of the Skin

Terminology of skin disorders

Dermatologists use very specific terms to describe skin lesions (local involvement) and eruptions (widespread involvement). These terms are split into macroscopic and microscopic.

Macroscopic appearances
Macule
A macule is an area of color or textural change (Fig. 8.1, A); macules are seen in vitiligo (hypopigmentation), freckles (hyperpigmentation), and capillary hemangioma (erythematous). They are flat lesions.

Papule
A papule is a solid elevation of skin less than 5 mm in diameter (Fig. 8.1, B). Papules can appear in various guises: dome-shaped (xanthomas), flat-topped (lichen planus), or spicular (accompanying hair follicles).

Nodule
A nodule is an elevation greater than 5 mm in diameter that may be either solid or edematous (Fig. 8.1, C). Nodules are seen in rheumatoid arthritis, and a dermatofibroma is an example of the lesion.

Plaque
A plaque is an extended papule, palpable as a plateau-like elevation of skin no more than 5 mm in elevation but in general measuring more than 2 cm in diameter (Fig. 8.1, D). Plaques are commonly seen in psoriasis and mycosis fungoides infection.

Vesicle
Less than 5 mm in diameter, a vesicle is a skin blister filled with clear fluid (Fig. 8.1, E). Vesicles may be subepidermal or intraepidermal, and they may be singular or grouped.

Pustule
Similar to a vesicle, a pustule is filled with a visible collection of pus rather than free fluid and may, but not always, indicate an infection (Fig. 8.1, F). A furuncle is an example of an infected pustule, while the pustules that appear in psoriasis are sterile.

Bulla
A bulla is a vesicle that is greater than 5 mm in diameter (Fig. 8.1, G). Bullae occur in bulbous pemphigoid and pemphigus vulgaris.

Blister
Blisters are lesions of any size that are filled with clear fluid and form because of cleavage of the epidermis (Fig. 8.1, H). These may result from constant abrasion of the skin or from a pathologic process. The cleavage may be intraepidermal or subdermal.

Wheal
Wheals are transitory and consist of a compressible, red or white papule or plaque of edema (Fig. 8.1, I). They usually indicate urticaria.

Scale
Scales are flat flakes of abnormal skin that indicate disordered keratinocyte maturation and keratinization (Fig. 8.1, J). They vary in appearance, from large and polygonal-like fish scales in patients with ichthyosis to silvery and white flakes in patients with psoriasis.

Lichenification
Lichenification is a chronic thickening of the skin with increased skin markings; the condition is caused by constant rubbing or scratching.

Excoriation
An excoriation is a superficial linear abrasion caused by scratching.

Onycholysis
Onycholysis is the separation of the nail from the nail bed, leading to the nail plate becoming thickened, crumbly, and yellow. Subungual hyperkeratosis subsequently occurs. This condition is associated with many disorders, including psoriasis, fungal infections, and trauma.

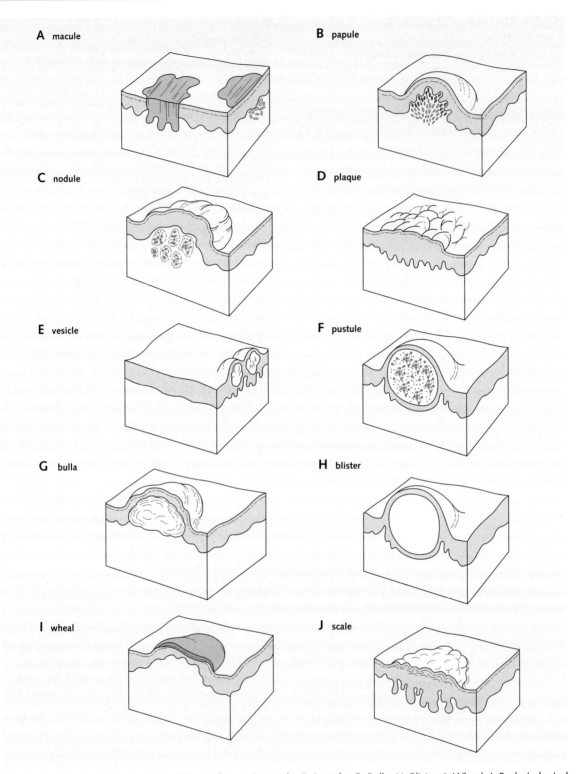

Fig. 8.1 A. Macule. B. Papule. C. Nodule. D. Plaque. E. Vesicle. F. Pustule. G. Bulla. H. Blister. I. Wheal. J. Scale (adapted from *Dermatology: An Illustrated Color Text,* 2nd ed., by Gawkrodger DJ, Churchill Livingstone, 1997).

Microscopic appearances

Hyperkeratosis

Hyperkeratosis is hypertrophy of the cornified layer of the skin, which leads to thickening of the epidermis.

Parakeratosis

Parakeratosis is a pathologic process in which the nuclei of the cells in the stratum corneum persist. It is associated with disease states such as psoriasis.

Acanthosis

Acanthosis is hypertrophy of the stratum spinosum of the epidermis.

Dyskeratosis

Dyskeratosis describes a process in which keratinocytes mature early, becoming keratinized before they reach the surface of the skin. Cells in the epidermis become rounded and may break away from other cells.

Acantholysis

Acantholysis is a pathologic process whereby the prickle cells of the stratum spinosum separate, leading to atrophy of the epidermis. Acantholysis is seen in diseases such as pemphigus vulgaris and keratosis follicularis.

Papillomatosis

Papillomatosis is a term used to describe diseases characterized by a number of papillomas.

Lentiginous

Lentiginous describes skin that is covered by lentigines: brown macules that resemble freckles, except with the regular border and rete (ridges that freckles lack).

Spongiosis

Spongiosis is an inflammatory intercellular edema of the epidermis.

Exocytosis

Exocytosis describes a process whereby material is released into extracellular space by fusion of an intracellular membrane-bound vesicle.

Erosion

Erosion is a destructive lesion of the skin that affects only the epidermis and that heals without scarring.

Ulceration

Ulceration refers to the formation of an ulcer, which is a lesion on the skin's surface that is formed by sloughing of inflammatory, necrotic tissue.

Inflammation and skin eruptions

Psoriasis

Psoriasis is an inflammatory dermatosis with a chronic course. It is presents with erythematous, well-demarcated, silvery-scaled plaques.

Classification of types

There are six different variants of psoriasis: plaque, flexural, palmoplantar pustulosis, guttate, scalp, and acrodermatitis of Hallopeau (Fig. 8.2).

Plaque

Plaque is the most commonly seen type of psoriasis. Well-defined red plaques topped with silvery-white scales are usually seen over the extensor surfaces of the limbs (i.e., elbows and knees), with smaller lesions over the limbs and trunk (Plate 1). The plaque discs can be large or small and may itch.

Flexural

The lesions in flexural psoriasis are clearly demarcated, pink and glazed, and lack the scales of plaque arthritis. The sites normally affected include the groin, perianal regions, and genital skin. Less commonly, the inframammary skin folds and the umbilicus may be affected.

Palmoplantar pustulosis

This type of pustular psoriasis affects the palms of the hands and soles of the feet. The sterile pustules, which are related in severity to disease activity, can appear white, yellow, or brown when dried. When accompanied by universal scaling on the trunk and limbs (erythrodermic psoriasis), pustular psoriasis is known as generalized pustular psoriasis, which is a serious and potentially fatal condition. This serious condition is seen either spontaneously or after administration of potent oral or topical corticosteroids, and it involves treatment and problems similar to that of widespread burn management. Palmoplantar pustulosis usually affects cigarette-smoking, middle-aged women; some of these women have also been diagnosed with classic plaque psoriasis.

137

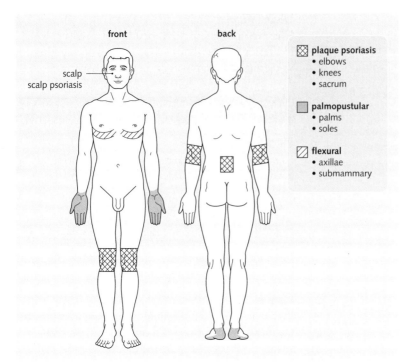

front   back

plaque psoriasis
• elbows
• knees
• sacrum

palmopustular
• palms
• soles

flexural
• axillae
• submammary

scalp
scalp psoriasis

Fig. 8.2 Distribution of the different types of psoriasis.

Guttate

Guttate psoriasis is characterized by "drop-like" eruptions that appear symmetrically on the trunk and limbs. This type of psoriasis may follow a streptococcal throat infection and is more common in young adults.

Scalp

Scalp psoriasis may often be the only clinical sign of psoriasis. Hyperkeratized plaques can be seen at the hair margin; the scales appear thicker and are better demarcated than dandruff.

Acrodermatitis of Hallopeau

Although the nails are affected by psoriasis in half of all individuals who have been diagnosed with this condition, acrodermatitis of Hallopeau is a rare, indolent (inactive) variant that only affects the fingers and nails.

Epidemiology

About 2% of the Western world suffers from psoriasis; it is less common in Asia and Africa. The male:female ratio is 1:1, and the disease commonly presents in the second and third decade, although onset may occur at any age. It is rare in children aged 8 years and under.

Etiology

Psoriasis has a strong genetic link, with identical twin studies showing a concordance of 80%, and 35% of patients showing a family history. The inheritance is polygenic; HLA antigens CW6, B13, and B17 have strong correlations with the disorder, and environmental factors are thought to trigger the disease. Drugs such as β-blockers, lithium, and antimalarials may precipitate the disorder or make existing psoriasis worse. Trauma to the upper layers of the skin, such as a scratch or a surgical scar, may lead to the formation of psoriatic skin at the site of damage: this is termed the Koebner phenomenon (Plate 2). Sunlight aggravates psoriasis in 10% of individuals; however, exposure to sunlight is beneficial for most.

Pathology

Active, psoriatic skin has a cell turnover rate that is 20–30 times faster than that of normal skin. The epidermal turnover time dramatically decreases from the normal 30 days to 3–4 days. Because of the increase in cell production, acanthosis results and manifests as the scaly plaque of psoriasis. Parakeratosis also occurs (Fig. 8.3).

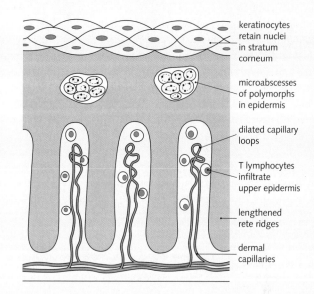

keratinocytes
retain nuclei
in stratum
corneum

microabscesses
of polymorphs
in epidermis

dilated capillary
loops

T lymphocytes
infiltrate
upper epidermis

lengthened
rete ridges

dermal
capillaries

Fig. 8.3 Histologic changes in psoriasis.

Complications
Erythroderma
Classified as inflammatory dermatosis that involves more than 90% of the skin surface, erythroderma needs prompt hospital admission because the systemic complications can be fatal. Erythrodermic psoriasis can be precipitated by the withdrawal of steroid treatment or an intercurrent drug eruption.

Psoriatic arthritis
About 5% of patients with psoriasis develop a joint disease. A distal arthritis that causes swelling of toes and digits (called dactylitis) is the most common form, but a rheumatoid-like arthritis with a similar polyarthritic pattern may also develop. Severe psoriasis may cause mutilans arthropathy, a destructive arthritis that erodes the small bones of the hands and feet, leading to progressive deformity. In addition, patients with psoriasis who are HLA B27-positive may develop ankylosing spondylitis.

Bacterial infection
Although a bacterial infection is rare, staphylococci can infect psoriatic plaques.

Management
The management of psoriasis is split into topical and systemic treatments. Topical treatments are usually the first line of treatment; systemic therapy is used for psoriasis that is not responsive to topical treatment, for psoriasis of life-threatening severity, or psoriasis that severely restricts the patient's quality of life.

Topical
Tar-based preparations: These treatments are distilled from coal tar and are frequently used for inpatient care. Often combined with ultraviolet B (UVB) exposure or dithranol (anthralin; see next paragraph), the tar preparations appear to work by altering the DNA synthesis of the skin. The disadvantages of this treatment are that the tar preparations stain the skin, can cause a burning sensation, and have a strong odor.

Dithranol (anthralin): A messy and smelly treatment, administration of dithranol interferes with skin mitosis. Lassar's paste is the most common preparation of dithranol used in hospitals, and it is applied over psoriatic plaques. Because normal skin is irritated by the preparation, surrounding skin can be protected by the application of white paraffin (e.g.,

139

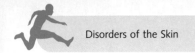
Vaseline). The dithranol only needs to be applied to the skin for 30 minutes per day—under this regime, the psoriasis will usually clear up within 3 weeks.

Vitamin D analogues: Topical synthetic vitamin D analogues inhibit cell proliferation and promote keratinocyte differentiation, thus reversing some of the structural abnormalities of the skin present in psoriasis. The analogues have a similar efficacy to dithranol.

Topical corticosteroids: Use of topical corticosteroids should be considered only for stubborn plaques or for the treatment of lesions on the face, genitals, or flexures, because the steroids are nonirritating. Topical steroids are available as creams, ointment, lotion, and gels (for scalp). Their use must be strictly monitored, because the side effects caused by steroid usage include:
- Atrophy of the skin.
- Induction of acne or perioral dermatitis.
- Precipitation of unstable psoriasis upon treatment withdrawal.
- Allergic contact dermatitis.
- Infection (fungal, bacterial, or viral) precipitated by steroidal treatment.
- Reduced efficacy after prolonged use (tachyphylaxis).
- Systemic effects of steroidal treatment—growth retardation, cushingoid appearance, and endocrine effects caused by systemic absorption of steroid.

Salicylic acid ointment: This ointment is used to treat psoriasis of the scalp, palms, and hands. The scalp can also be treated with a coconut oil compound or a tar-containing shampoo.

Systemic therapy
Methotrexate: This drug acts by inhibiting cell mitosis; it is usually administered orally, although it can be given intramuscularly or intravenously. Contraindications include a history of alcoholism, liver disease, peptic ulceration, colitis, pregnancy, and acute infection; normal liver, kidney, and marrow function must be established before the treatment begins, and the patient must be monitored carefully throughout the course of the treatment. The most serious side effects of methotrexate include hepatic fibrosis and cirrhosis. Results are usually observed within 2–4 weeks.

Retinoids: Acitretin, a vitamin A analogue, can be used to treat both plaque and pustular psoriasis. It may also be used as a topical treatment or may be combined with UVB or psoralens and high-intensity ultraviolet A (PUVA) therapy. Acitretin is teratogenic; if given to women of child-bearing age, effective contraception must be started 1 month before beginning treatment and continued throughout the treatment period; the patient must also take contraception for 3 years after stopping the course due to the long half-life of the drug.

Cyclosporin: This immunosuppressant clears psoriasis when taken in high doses. It is nephrotoxic, however, and renal function should be carefully monitored throughout the course of administration. The long-term effects of taking cyclosporin are not yet known.

Fumaric acid derivatives: Although the short-term effectiveness of these drugs is good, 75% of patients on this treatment complain of acute side effects, including gastrointestinal symptoms and flushing. Many patients therefore stop taking the drug; there is also no evidence to support use in long-term maintenance treatment.

Eczema and contact dermatitis
Definitions
Eczema and contact dermatitis are used interchangeably to describe the same condition—a noninfective inflammatory condition.

Atopic eczema (dermatitis)
Etiology
Atopic eczema often occurs in patients with a medical or family history of asthma, hay fever, or conjunctivitis and affects about 10–15% of children in North America. An atopic family history (the inherited tendency to develop asthma, atopic eczema, or hay fever) is positive in 65% of patients; 60% of those likely to present with atopy will do so in the first year of life. In 75% of patients, the disorder will remit by the age of 15 years.

Pathogenesis
High levels of circulating IgE antibodies, coupled with defective T cell function, are thought to cause reactions to commonly encountered allergens such as house dust mites. The resulting inflammation is pruritic and affects both the dermis and the epidermis (Fig. 8.4).

Clinical features
Atopic eczema usually presents in the first 6 months of life as a symmetrical erythematous eruption affecting the face, trunk, and limbs (Plate 3). As the child reaches 2 years, the eruption increasingly

A acute

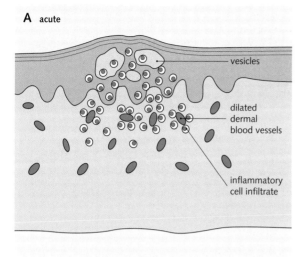

- vesicles
- dilated dermal blood vessels
- inflammatory cell infiltrate

B chronic

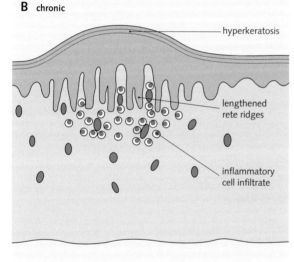

- hyperkeratosis
- lengthened rete ridges
- inflammatory cell infiltrate

Fig. 8.4 Histologic changes in eczema (adapted from *Dermatology: An Illustrated Color Text,* 2nd ed., by Gawkrodger DJ, Churchill Livingstone, 1997).

affects the flexures (Fig. 8.5). Lichenification, excoriations, and dry skin occur, all of which are aggravated by the child scratching or rubbing the affected skin. The pruritus may affect sleep.

Management

Conservative management: Educating the patient and family is important in the management of atopic eczema: the good prognosis should be stressed. Various lifestyle changes can be undertaken to lessen skin irritation: loose-fitting cotton clothing, avoidance of heat and irritants (e.g., wool and, in adults, job-related substances), trimming down of nails to avoid excessive scratching.

If pets are thought to aggravate the disease, provisions should be made, and efforts to minimize the presence of house dust mites can be helpful. Similarly, if a history suggesting a food allergy is given, the offending food should be avoided. Both local and national support groups exist for patients with atopic eczema; details of both should be made available to the patient.

Topical therapy

Emollients: Aqueous cream, emulsifying ointment, and bath oil emollients moisturize the skin, which in turn lessen the pruritus.

Topical steroids: Because of the side effects of topical steroids, hydrocortisone ointment should be started at the lowest potency and gradually increased in strength until an effective dose is found. It should be applied twice a day.

Antibiotics and antiseptics: These are used to treat the infective complications of eczema; bacterial (usually *Staphylococcus aureus*) and viral (viral warts, molluscum contagiosum, or herpes simplex) infection may exacerbate the disorder. Eczema infected with herpes simplex is termed eczema herpeticum.

Medicated bandages: Bandages impregnated with coal tar or ichthammol paste that are left on overnight may be useful in excoriated or lichenified eczema. With exudative eczema, nonmedicated wet dressings may help.

Systemic therapy

Antihistamines: Sedative antihistamines (diphenhydramine elixir, 25–50 mg) given at night may decrease the need to scratch.

Oral antibiotics and antiviral agents: Penicillinase-resistant penicillin or cephalosporin is often given to treat the secondary infection of eczema eruptions. Inpatient treatment with the antiviral acyclovir is used to manage eczema herpeticum.

Other systemic treatments: Severe and resistant eczema can be treated by PUVA or a 6-week course of cyclosporin.

Contact dermatitis

Eczema precipitated by an exogenous substance is termed contact dermatitis. Clinically similar to atopic eczema, it is caused by skin irritants rather

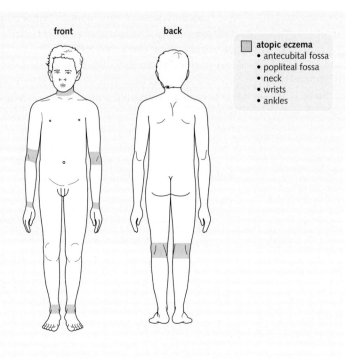

front   back

atopic eczema
• antecubital fossa
• popliteal fossa
• neck
• wrists
• ankles

Fig. 8.5 Distribution of eczema.

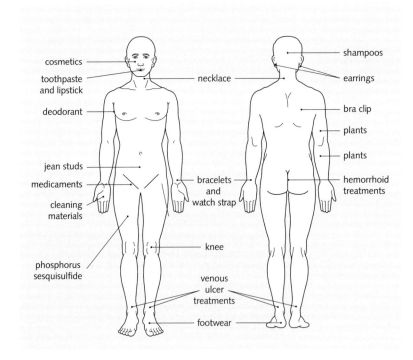

cosmetics

toothpaste
and lipstick

deodorant

jean studs

medicaments

cleaning
materials

phosphorus
sesquisulfide

necklace

bracelets
and
watch strap

knee

venous
ulcer
treatments

footwear

shampoos

earrings

bra clip

plants

plants

hemorrhoid
treatments

Fig. 8.6 Distribution of contact dermatitis. (Note that medical ointments and creams may cause rashes wherever applied) (redrawn from *Dermatology: An Illustrated Color Text*, 2nd ed., by Gawkrodger DJ, Churchill Livingstone, 1997).

that allergens and is a major cause of illness in industrial settings (Plate 4). Atopic patients are more prone to development of contact dermatitis.

The site of presentation may give a clue to the causative factors of contact dermatitis (Fig. 8.6). The most important skin irritants include chemicals,

142

solvents, detergents, abrasives, and even water; the most common allergy is to nickel, which affects 1 in 10 women and 1 in a 100 men. Patch testing is useful in determining the irritant involved, and management is largely based on subsequently avoiding it once identified. Topical steroids are the secondary line of treatment.

Other forms of dermatitis
The other forms of endogenous dermatitis are listed in Fig. 8.7.

Urticaria and angioedema
Urticaria and angioedema are two conditions associated with acute edema. Urticaria, commonly known as hives, is characterized by transient, pruritic wheals that are caused by extravascular plasma leakage in the dermis; angioedema is a more widespread collection of extravascular fluid that involves the dermis and subcutaneous tissue (superficial fascia subcutis).

Pathology
The lesions arise from the release of histamine and various other substances caused by mast cell degranulation. This release is mediated through one of several pathways: IgE-mediated (type I) sensitivity, complement activation, direct release (usually drug-related), or blocking of the prostaglandin pathway (caused by drugs such as aspirin and nonsteroidal anti-inflammatory drugs [NSAIDs]).

Clinical features
About 75% of urticaria cases are classified as chronic, idiopathic, or acute. Wheals rapidly appear and disappear on the skin, usually within 24 hours, and leave no residual mark. The lesions vary in size, shape, and number and may be accompanied by angioedema of the tongue and lips. Often no underlying cause is found, and the disorder usually spontaneously resolves within a few months. With acute cases, the onset can usually be traced to an allergen that provokes a sudden IgE-mediated (type I) hypersensitivity reaction.

Management
Investigations should be instigated to detect provoking factors if the cause remains unclear after the history and examination. Dermographism

Endogenous forms of dermatitis	
Type of dermatitis	**Comments**
Seborrheic dermatitis	Disease of adults; *Pityrosporum ovale* plays an important role; dry, persistent redness and scaling seen on face; pruritis ani and chronic otitis externa are common symptoms
Venous dermatitis of legs	Feature of chronic venous insufficiency in legs; caused by venous hypertension in deep veins owing to valvular incompetence
Hand dermatitis	Includes pompholyx, a vesicular pattern of dermatitis; may also be caused by discoid dermatitis, primary irritant hand dermatitis, allergic contact dermatitis, and hyperkeratotic eczema
Asteatotic dermatitis	Seen mainly in older adults, particularly in the winter, and usually on the legs; consists of fine scaling, minor erythema, and superficial fissuring
Neurodermatitis	Localized lichenification seen in adult women on occipital scalp, nape, neck, and arms; lesions are well-defined ovoid or elongated plaques; hyperpigmentation is common; itching intermittent and intense
Discoid dermatitis	Multiple, well-defined discoid lesions with prominent edema; may be atopic or may be precipitated by emotional stress
Generalized exfoliative dermatitis	Also known as erythroderma; skin is erythematous, edematous and scaly; may be complicated by reversible loss of body hair; disease tends to be self-limiting

Fig. 8.7 Other endogenous forms of dermatitis.

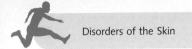

(wheals induced by firm stroking of the skin, a condition that is present in 5% of the population) can be demonstrated, and cold urticaria can be induced by applying ice to the skin for 1 minute. Hereditary angioedema can be detected by a low serum level of C_1 esterase inhibitor.

The mainstay of treatment is the use of antihistamines (e.g., diphenhydramine, hydroxyline, cyproheptadine), although management should also involve the avoidance of provoking factors. Systemic steroids may be used to treat severe acute angioedema but not the chronic version. Acute anaphylactic shock or airway obstruction (caused by angioedema) should be treated immediately with a 1-mg injection of adrenaline—this treatment saves lives.

Lichenoid eruptions
Lichen planus
Lichen planus is a fairly common disorder that affects the flexor surfaces, mucous membranes, and genitalia. It presents as pruritic, papular violaceous lesions that may coalesce to form small plaques (Plate 5). A white lace-like pattern may form on the top of plaques; this is called Wickham's striae. Lichen planus may also present as annular, atrophic (rare), bullous, or follicular lesions. Half of all patients recover spontaneously within 9 months, but in some, the lesions may persist for up to 18 months. Although the disease is self-limiting, symptomatic treatment involves the use of topical steroids or PUVA in resistant cases.

Lichen sclerosus
Characterized by white, lichenoid, and atrophic lesions that appear on the genitalia, lichen sclerosus is an immune-associated disorder that has a male: female ratio of 1:10. It is an uncommon disorder that usually presents in middle age. Management of genital lichen sclerosus involves topical steroids, with an antiseptic or antibiotic if necessary. Nongenital lichen sclerosus does not require treatment.

Lichen nitidus
Lichen nitidus is a rare lichenoid eruption that features tiny monomorphic papules; these contain a lymphocytic infiltrate that causes the expansion of single dermal papillae, visible under microscopy. The condition is asymptomatic and requires no treatment.

Papulosquamous eruptions
Pityriasis rosea
A pityriasis rosea eruption is usually preceded by a "herald patch"—a single erythematous oval macule that appears 4–14 days before the generalized eruption of multiple, smaller plaques over the trunk, upper arms, and thighs. The rash is symmetrical and may follow the distribution of the ribs, forming a "Christmas tree" pattern.

Individual lesions are either "medallion" plaques (oval, rose-colored patches that are slightly raised around the edges and that may have a fine collar of scales) or maculopapules (Plate 6). Pityriasis rosea usually affects those aged between 15 and 40 years; it is uncommon to be affected by a second eruption after the first clears up. It usually takes 1–2 months for the skin to heal. The etiology of the disease is unclear, but is thought to be viral in origin. Lesions may be pruritic; the itch can be relieved by a mild topical steroid. Since the eruption is self-limiting, no other treatment is required.

Tinea versicolor
Otherwise known as pityriasis versicolor, this disorder is caused by fungal infection. It presents as irregular brown or pinkish macules that coalesce to form larger, superficially scaly lesions. Eruption sites include the neck, shoulders, upper arms, and upper trunk.

Tinea versicolor mostly affects young adults and is more common in tropical climates. Examination under Wood's light shows skin fluorescence, and, under microscopy, skin scrapings demonstrate the spores and short, rod-like hyphae, which is the so-called "grapes and bananas" appearance. The management involves application of a topical imidazole antifungal treatment with 2.5% selenium sulfide or involves taking an oral ketoconazole for resistant cases. If hypopigmentation changes have occurred in darker skin, the patient should be warned that this discoloration may take some time to heal.

Reiter's disease
Reiter's disease refers to a collection of physical signs, which include polyarthropathy, urethritis, iritis, and psoriasiform eruption. The disease affects HLA B27-positive men and usually follows a nongonococcal urethritis or bowel infection. The skin lesions occurring in Reiter's disease include keratoderma blennorrhagicum and balanitis of the penis. Joint arthropathy and nail involvement may be

severe. Management involves treating the initial infection, administering anti-inflammatory analgesia for the joint, and using topical steroids for skin lesions.

Parapsoriasis

Also known as chronic superficial dermatitis, parapsoriasis is an eruption of pink, oval, or round plaques that are topped by scales. The lesions may be premalignant. They appear in mid-adulthood to late adulthood and are usually found on the abdomen, buttocks, or thighs. Some lesions progress to malignant, cutaneous T cell lymphomas (mycosis fungoides), although the majority of lesions remain benign. Biopsy is necessary to detect premalignant plaques; treatment is with topical steroids for benign parapsoriasis and PUVA or UVB for premalignant plaques.

Photodermatoses
Idiopathic causes
Polymorphic light eruption

The most common of the photodermatoses, polymorphic light eruption dermatitis (of variable severity) features pruritic, urticarial papules, plaques, and vesicles that appear on the skin 24 hours after exposure to the light. Sunscreen is used as a protective measure and a course of PUVA exposure at the close of spring can often acclimatize the skin, so a patient will not suffer light-induced problems during the summer months.

Chronic actinic dermatitis

Also known as actinic reticuloid dermatitis, chronic actinic dermatitis is a rare disorder that affects men in mid-adulthood to late adulthood. It is characterized by the development of thick, lichenified plaques on sun-exposed skin, and the patient may have a previous history of contact dermatitis or photodermatitis. The condition is managed by avoidance of the precipitating sunlight, use of protective sunscreen, and treatment with topical steroids. If the dermatitis is resistant to these measures, administration of oral steroids or azathioprine may be necessary.

Solar urticaria and actinic prurigo

In solar urticaria, skin wheals appear within minutes of exposure to sunlight and clear within 1–2 hours. With actinic prurigo, sun-induced papules and lichenified nodules first appear in childhood and may resolve by adolescence. Both conditions are rare.

Other causes

Other causes of photodermatoses include:
- Porphyria—metabolite accumulation due to enzyme insufficiency.
- Pellagra—nicotinic acid deficiency.
- Genetic—e.g., xeroderma pigmentosum.
- Drug-induced—e.g., nifedipine, thiazides, angiotensin-converting enzyme inhibitors, and NSAIDs.

Effects of sunlight on other dermatologic conditions

Sunlight aggravates the following conditions:
- Lupus erythematosus.
- Facial herpes simplex.
- Rosacea.
- Psoriatic disease (a minority).
- Vitiligo.

It benefits the following conditions:
- Acne.
- Psoriasis.
- Parapsoriasis.
- Pityriasis rosea.
- Atopic eczema.

Infection and infestation

Bacterial infections
The normal skin microflora

Normal bacteria resident on the skin include staphylococci, micrococci, corynebacteria, and propionibacteria. In addition to bacteria, other microorganisms that are present in healthy skin include yeasts and mites. The numbers of microorganisms vary depending on the site (e.g., forearm versus moist environs of axillae) and the individual.

Diseases caused by overgrowth of normal flora
Erythrasma

An overgrowth of normal commensals can lead to erythrasma, a dry, red, scaly eruption that usually affects the skin folds; the affected skin will fluoresce under a Wood's light. Erythrasma will clear up when treated with imidazole cream, topical fusidic acid, or oral erythromycin or tetracycline.

Trichomycosis axillaris

Trichomycosis refers to the yellowish substance formed on axillary hair as a result of corynebacteria

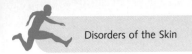

overgrowth. Antimicrobial cream will usually clear the problem.

Pitted keratolysis

A proliferation of micrococci on the foot, encouraged by tight-fitting footwear and sweaty feet, may lead to foul-smelling, discolored, and pitted nails—micrococci can destroy the nail's keratin—called pitted keratolysis. Better hygiene will limit the problem, and topical neomycin or a 0.01% aqueous potassium permanganate foot soak may also help.

Staphylococcal infections

Impetigo

Impetigo can be caused by staphylococcus or streptococcus infection. It presents as superficial skin blisters, which are easily ruptured to leave a crusted yellow exudate (Plate 7). The lesions are highly contagious and spread rapidly; they may complicate other skin disorders, such as atopic eczema and herpes simplex. Management involves removing the residual crusts by soaking them in saline. If the infection becomes generalized, systemic antibiotics are necessary. For the most serious form of impetigo (caused by *Streptococcus pyogenes*), oral penicillinase-resistant penicillin, cloxacillin, or a first-generation cephalosporin is given to the patient to prevent glomerulonephritic complications.

Ecthyma

Ecthyma results from the growth of staphylococci in the skin of debilitated, immunosuppressed, or diabetic patients after minor trauma. The bacterial infection leads to development of a number of shallow (and occasionally deep) round ulcers, usually on the legs. The ulcers leave scarring upon healing after treatment with systemic and topical antibiotics.

Folliculitis

Caused by infection with *S. aureus* or gram-negative bacteria, folliculitis results from the pustular infection of multiple hair follicles. The pustules have erythematous edges and often contain an emerging hair shaft. Management is with topical and systemic antibiotics; to prevent recurrence, the patient should be educated about improved personal hygiene.

Scalded skin syndrome

Scalded skin syndrome is a serious condition, usually caused by an autoimmune response to specific strains of staphylococcus infection. It usually affects infants and causes severe erythema and the shedding of large sheets of epidermis from the body. The disorder responds well to prompt treatment with floxacillin or erythromycin, although a drug-induced adult variant of the condition (toxic epidermal necrolysis) is often fatal.

Streptococcal infections

Erysipelas

Presenting with localized erythema, swelling, and tenderness, erysipelas is an acute infection of the dermis, caused by *S. pyogenes*. The inflammation is well-defined and may have palpable borders. The eruption follows a general malaise, with flu-like symptoms.

In healthy individuals, the eruptions clear in 2–3 weeks after treatment with oral penicillin to prevent streptococcal septicemia. Penicillin can also be used prophylactically with recurrent attacks, which lead to lymphatic damage and irreversible edema. Resistant cases should be treated with cloxacillin or cephalexin.

Necrotizing fasciitis

Necrotizing fasciitis is a serious infection that may occur after minor trauma; progress is often fulminant and it must be treated immediately to prevent serious skin necrosis in the affected area. It is usually caused by group A β-hemolytic streptococci. The infection is characterized by a high fever and an ill-defined erythema that usually occurs on the leg. Superficial fascia and underlying muscle tissue are rapidly destroyed. Systemic antibiotics and surgical debridement of the resultant necrotic tissue aid recovery.

Mycobacterial infections

Lupus vulgaris

The most common *Mycobacterium tuberculosis* skin infection, lupus vulgaris, arises as a postprimary infection and usually begins in childhood. Over time, initially painless, red-brown nodules coalesce to form larger plaques, most commonly seen on the head and neck. Complications include the destruction of deeper skin tissues and the development of squamous cell carcinoma in long-standing lesions. A biopsy will aid the diagnosis, and the Mantoux test will usually be positive. Treatment is with a three-drug program, usually rifampicin, isoniazid, and pyrazinamide. After an 8-week course, the pyrazinamide is stopped, and the other drugs are continued for 6–9 months depending on the response.

Scrofuloderma

Scrofuloderma is an infection that occurs on the skin superficial to a lymph node affected with tuberculosis or an affected bone or joint. A dull red nodule develops and ulcerates, which can lead to fistulas, granulation, and scarring.

Warty tuberculosis

Warty tuberculosis results from the inoculation of tuberculosis into the skin of previously infected patients. It forms warty plaques on the hands, knees, and buttocks; the condition is now extremely rare in the Western world but is still common in developing countries.

Spirochetal infections
Secondary syphilis

The secondary stage of syphilis begins 1–3 months after the primary chancre and is characterized by pink or copper-colored papules that appear on the trunk, palms, limbs, and soles. If left untreated, the papules will resolve in 1–3 months.

Yaws, bejel, and pinta

Yaws, bejel, and pinta are nonvenereal treponemal infections that are endemic in tropical developing countries. In all three, the serology is positive for syphilis, and the infection may be treated with benzathine penicillin G.

Lyme disease

Lyme disease is caused by *Borrelia burgdorferi* and is spread by tick bites. Lyme disease is characterized by a slowly expanding erythematous ring at the site of the initial tick bite. Complications include arthritis, neurologic pathology, and cardiac problems; administration of oral doxycycline, penicillin G, tetracycline, or amoxicillin is normally a successful treatment.

Other bacterial infections
Anthrax

Primarily an animal disease, anthrax causes hemorrhagic bullae at the site of inoculation. The lesion is accompanied by edema and fever. The diagnosis is by culture of the blister fluid, and the disease is treated by intramuscular injections of procaine penicillin G or intravenous procaine penicillin G combined with streptomycin (followed by oral administration).

Gram-negative infections

Gram-negative bacilli, such as *Pseudomonas aeruginosa*, may infect skin wounds such as leg ulcers. They may also cause nail discoloration, folliculitis, and cellulitis (Plate 8).

Viral infections
Viral warts

Also known as verrucae, viral warts are benign cutaneous tumors caused by infection with human papilloma virus (HPV). The virus spreads through direct contact, sexual contact, and also through water (e.g., local swimming pools). There are over 50 HPV subtypes, with different types being responsible for specific lesions: hand warts, plantar warts, genital warts, and other such conditions.

Common warts appear as dome-shaped papules with a papilliferous surface (Plate 9). Between 30 and 50% of common warts resolve spontaneously within 6 months; hand and foot warts can be treated with an abrasive stone or scalpel to pare down keratotic skin to allow easier treatment with drugs, cryotherapy, and cautery.

Molluscum contagiosum

Caused by a DNA poxvirus, molluscum contagiosum mainly affects children and teenagers. The lesions appear as multiple pearly pink umbilicated papules, a few millimeters in diameter, that spread through direct contact or through a medium such as towels. They commonly occur on the face, neck, and trunk and are treated by expressing the "cheesy" contents through forceps pressure, curettage, or cryotherapy. Because this treatment can be painful, with young children it is easier to teach a parent how to squeeze the affected lesions after a warm bath to soften the skin.

Herpes simplex

A common infection, caused by herpesvirus hominis, herpes simplex has two types of primary infection. Type 1 primary infection is facial or nongenital and is sometimes accompanied by fever, malaise, lymphadenopathy, and occasionally gingivostomatitis. If symptomatic, the illness lasts 2 weeks.

Type 2 primary infection occurs after sexual contact in young adults; lesions develop on the vulva, vagina, penis, or in the perianal region. If the infection occurs in pregnant women, it is an indication for cesarean delivery; neonatal infection with herpes simplex is commonly fatal.

After the initial attack, the virus becomes latent, residing in the dorsal root ganglion. Reactivation leads

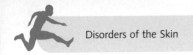
to lesions at a similar site each time, often manifesting on the lips, face, or genitals. The vesicular eruption may be preceded by a tingling or burning; crusts form within 1–2 days, and the lesions clear after a week.

Treatment involves the use of acyclovir, idoxuridine, or trifluridine cream, with more severe infections requiring the use of systemic acyclovir or vidarabine. Treatment of genital herpes can also include the use of famciclovir; barrier contraception should be used by those infected, and sexual intercourse should be avoided altogether during symptomatic episodes of the disease.

Herpes zoster

Otherwise known as shingles, this infection occurs in a dermatomal distribution and follows a previous infection with the varicella-zoster (chickenpox) virus. Reactivation of the virus leads to a self-limiting, vesicular eruption accompanied by local lymphadenopathy, pain numbness, and paresthesia. The thoracic dermatomes are most often involved (Plate 10) although involvement of the ophthalmic division of the trigeminal nerve is common in older adults and may result in corneal ulcers.

Treatment involves taking analgesics and applying calamine lotion to dry the lesions. If a secondary bacterial infection occurs, topical antiseptics or antibiotics are necessary. Severe cases require oral or systemic acyclovir.

Fungal infections

Human fungal infections are called mycoses: they are classified into superficial, cutaneous infections (tinea, candidosis, and pityriasis versicolor) and deep, systemic infections (e.g., actinomycosis, sporotrichosis, and blastomycosis).

Dermatophyte infections

Fungi of dermatophyte infections reproduce by producing spores: they cause tinea infection or "ringworm." The usual sites of dermatophyte infection are the nail, hair, and stratum corneum of the skin. There are three different types of dermatophyte that cause tinea in humans: *Microsporum*, *Trichophyton*, and *Epidermophyton*.

Microsporum

Infecting skin and hair, *Microsporum* fluoresce under a Wood's light and usually cause infection during childhood. Along with *Trichophyton* fungi, they cause tinea capitis (ringworm of the scalp). Two *Microsporum* are responsible: *M. audouini*, which spreads from child to child and is responsible for epidemics in schools, and *M. canis*, which is passed on from family pets, mainly kittens and puppies.

Trichophyton

Trichophyton causes many types of tinea; this type of dermatophyte spore cannot be detected by a Wood's light and requires examination of skin scrapings under microscopy for diagnosis. The most common example is *T. rubrum*, which causes tinea cruris (groin), tinea pedis (foot), tinea barbae (beard), tinea faciei (glabrous skin of the face), as well as infection of the hands, feet, and nails.

Epidermophyton

Epidermophyton causes tinea cruris (ringworm of the groin) and tinea pedis (ringworm of the foot).

Candida albicans infections

Candida albicans is an opportunistic organism normally resident in the mouth and gastrointestinal tract. There are a number of predisposing factors that increase the risk of a *Candida albicans* infection:

- Pregnancy.
- Oral contraceptive pill.
- Wide-spectrum antibiotics.
- Corticosteroid treatment.
- Immunosuppressive drugs.
- Diabetes mellitus.
- Hypothyroidism.
- Blood dyscrasias.
- HIV infection.
- Poor hygiene.
- Humid environment.

Infection can occur as a genital, intertriginous, mucocutaneous, oral, paronychial, or systemic eruption. It usually presents as white plaques that can be itchy and sore (Plate 11). With systemic infection, red nodules can be seen in the skin. Management involves the cessation of systemic antibiotics if appropriate.

Topical therapy includes magenta paint and, more commonly, imidazoles. Amphotericin, nystatin, and miconazole are used for oral candida. Systemic therapy includes oral nystatin, ketoconazole, and fluconazole. Vaginal candida can be treated by a single dose of clotrimazole or econazole as a pessary.

Infestations
Insect bites

Insect bites can cause a chemical, irritated, or immune-mediated response in the skin caused by the introduction of foreign material into the body. Depending on the type of bite, the lesion can present as anything from itchy wheals to large bullae. Lesions are identified as insect bites by their pattern—either grouped or linear lesions that track up a limb. Secondary infection of the bite may occur.

Management involves elimination of the cause (e.g., bedbugs, cat fleas). Symptoms may be treated with hydrocortisone cream or calamine lotion.

Pediculosis (lice)

Lice infestations are of two types: pubic lice or body lice (Fig. 8.8). The latter is most common as head lice, which often cause epidemics in schools. Lice are spread by direct contact, and they lay eggs (nits) on hair. Body lice are found in individuals who are homeless or those who have poor hygiene and are spread through infested clothing or bedding. Pubic lice are generally found in young adults and are spread through sexual contact.

The lice cause itching, which can lead to excoriation of the skin and secondary infection. Management involves treatment with malathion, lindane, or carbaryl lotions, depending on the type of infestation.

Scabies

Caused by *Sarcoptes scabiei hominis*, a mite (Fig. 8.9) that can only survive on human skin, scabies infestation develops as a chronic and contagious disease that causes itching. The female mite burrows down into the skin at a rate of 2 mm a day, laying eggs as she goes. After 3 days, the eggs hatch, and they mature after 2 weeks. The mites mate; the males die, and the females continue the cycle.

The skin takes 4–6 weeks to react to the infestation, so the infection may be spread by direct contact before the problem is recognized. Burrows may be difficult to find, particularly when the disease has persisted for several weeks, because they are obscured by scratching and secondary lesions.

Clinical symptoms include excoriations caused by itching and scaly burrows measuring up to 1 cm in length, which are seen on the skin of infected

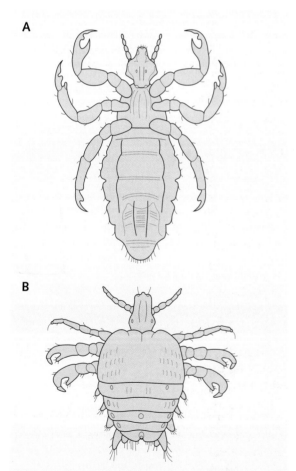

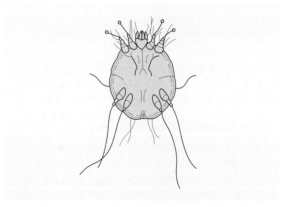

Fig. 8.8 A. Body louse (*Pediculus humanus*). B. Female pubic louse (adapted from *Dermatology: An Illustrated Color Text,* 2nd ed., by Gawkrodger DJ, Churchill Livingstone, 1997).

Fig. 8.9 Female scabies mite (adapted from *Dermatology: An Illustrated Color Text,* 2nd ed., by Gawkrodger DJ, Churchill Livingstone, 1997).

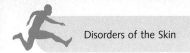

individuals (Plate 12). They are usually found on the wrists, ankles, nipples, and genitalia, and the mite may be visible at the end of the burrow as a small white dot. Extraction of the mite for microscopy from scrapings taken from the burrows confirms the diagnosis.

In institutions (e.g., nursing homes, hospitals) or in immunosuppressed patients, proliferation of the scabies mite leads to the formation of large, encrusted eruptions; this is known as "Norwegian scabies." Secondary infection is also common with scabies infestation. Management includes contact tracing and the use of lindane, malathion, and permethrin lotions to treat infected patients and contacts. Hydrocortisone, benzyl benzoate, and 10% sulfur ointment can also be used.

Tropical skin infections and infestations

Although not endemic in the Western world, tropical skin diseases can be seen in visitors and immigrants, and an awareness of the diseases listed in the upcoming paragraphs is useful for those who practice Western medicine.

Leprosy

Caused by *Mycobacterium leprae*, leprosy is spread via nasal droplets and takes several years to incubate. Depending on the degree of type IV hypersensitivity in an infected individual, the patient will develop either tuberculoid leprosy (strong cell-mediated immunity) or lepromatous leprosy (weak cell-mediated immunity). Tuberculoid leprosy affects peripheral nerves (anesthesia, muscle atrophy) and skin (red plaque facial lesions). Lepromatous leprosy mainly affects the skin, causing multiple symmetrical macules, papules, nodules, and plaques on the face (leonine facies), arms, legs, and buttocks.

Leprosy results in bone damage because of repeated trauma (tuberculoid) and saddle nose defect (lepromatous). If left untreated, ichthyosis, testicular atrophy, leg ulcers, acute skin lesions, and nerve destruction may result. Treatment lasts between 6 months and 2 years and involves use of rifampicin, dapsone, and clofazimine.

Leishmaniasis

Leishmaniasis is caused by a protozoon (*L. donovani*) transmitted to humans through the bite of sand flies. There are three types of leishmaniasis: cutaneous (endemic to the dry deserts around the Mediterranean), American (endemic to South and Central American tropics), and visceral (endemic to India). Treatment involves pentavalent antimony compounds and pentamidine.

Filariasis

Caused by the nematode worm *Wuchereria bancrofti*, filariasis is characterized by gross edema of the legs and scrotum and is termed elephantiasis. It is treated with diethylcarbamazine.

Larva migrans

Larva migrans is seen in patients who have recently traveled to tropical beaches, where they may have been infested with a hookworm larva. These larvae emerge from eggs present in the feces of infested cats and dogs; they penetrate the skin and migrate in a serpiginous fashion, causing intensely itchy red burrows. The disease is self-limiting because the larvae die within a few weeks; the condition, however, may be successfully treated with topical 10% thiabendazole cream or oral albendazole when the patient is symptomatic.

Onchocerciasis

Caused by *Onchocerca volvulus*, onchocerciasis is a filarial infestation common in Africa and South America where the filariae are transmitted through gnat bites. The adult worm may grow up to 7 cm long; microfilariae are found in the dermis and, more seriously, in the eye, causing blindness.

Granulomatous nodules are present on the skin, following an itchy, papular eruption. Onchocerciasis can be treated with a single dose of ivermectin, followed by repeated doses at 6-month intervals until the worm has been eradicated.

Tumors of the skin

Benign tumors of the skin
Epidermal tumors
Seborrheic wart

Otherwise known as basal cell papillomas, seborrheic warts are common, pigmented tumors of unknown etiology that affect older or middle-aged individuals. The tumor consists of basal keratinocytes. The warts are multiple or solitary and round or oval in shape, and they begin as small, lightly pigmented papules before becoming darkly pigmented, warty nodules that measure up to 6 cm in diameter (Plate 13).

The lesions appear to be stuck onto the skin and have well-defined margins and keratin plugs. They are found on the trunk and face and are usually treated by liquid nitrogen cryotherapy, curettage, or shave biopsy.

Skin tags

Skin tags are benign, pedunculated fibroepithelial polyps and are common lesions found in middle-aged to older adult patients. They are most commonly found in the neck, axillae, groin, and eyelids; if removal is required (usually on cosmetic grounds), the polyp stalk is cut and the lesion removed. Skin tags can also be removed by cryotherapy.

Epidermal cysts (keratinous cysts, sebaceous cysts)

Epidermal cysts are filled with keratin and arise from the epidermis or outer root of the hair follicle (pilar cyst). They are usually found on the scalp, face, and hands and are firm, mobile lesions that measure up to 3 cm in diameter. Excision will clear the lesion; bacterial infection may be a complication and may require antibiotics.

Milia

Milia are small (1–2 mm in size), keratin-filled, whitish, superficial cysts usually found or on the face or scrotum. They can appear at any age and may follow the healing of subepidermal blisters. They can be successfully excised using a sterile needle.

Dermal tumors
Dermatofibroma

Normally asymptomatic, dermatofibromas are common nodules present in the dermis that may or may not be pigmented. They usually occur on the legs and are more common in women than men. If the diagnosis is in doubt, an excisional biopsy should be performed.

Pyogenic granuloma

A pyogenic granuloma is an acquired hemangioma (despite the name, it is neither pyogenic nor granulomatous) that presents as a bright-red, blood-encrusted nodule on the finger, lip, foot, or face (Plate 14). The lesion, which develops rapidly over a few weeks, is pedunculated and bleeds easily. Pyogenic granuloma develops in children and young adults and is treated by excision. The excised material is examined histologically to exclude malignant melanoma.

Keloid

A keloid is a lesion arising from the excessive development of connective tissue that occurs after injury to the skin or inflammation. Unlike usual skin scarring, a keloid progresses beyond the limit of the original injury and presents as a hard nodule or plaque that is most commonly found on the upper back, chest, and ear lobes. Keloids are more common in the Afro-Caribbean population and are treated by steroid injections into the lesion.

Campbell-de-Morgan spot

Also known as cherry angiomas, Campbell-de-Morgan spots are capillary proliferations that present as bright-red papules in the middle-aged and older adult population. They are found on the trunk and can be excised by cauterization.

Lipomas

Lipomas present as soft subcutaneous masses found on the trunk, neck, and upper extremities. The fatty nodules may be multiple and are sometimes painful, in which case they can be removed by excision.

Nevi
Melanocytic nevi

Etiology: Commonly known as moles, melanocytic nevi are present in most Caucasian adults. The number of nevi appears to be influenced by a genetic component.

Pathology: The nevus cells are thought to derive from melanocytes, and histologically there are three different types of nevi (Fig. 8.10):
- Junctional—nevus cells cluster at the dermatoepithelial junction.
- Intradermal—nevus cells cluster in the dermis.
- Compound—nevus cells cluster at both sites.

Clinical features: Only congenital nevi are present at birth; other types develop during childhood and adolescence. Pregnancy or excessive sun exposure may cause the development of further nevi in later life. The number of melanocytic nevi present in Caucasians is usually between 10 and 30.

Complications: Dysplastic nevi that change size, shape, or color and those that itch or become inflamed or encrusted must be examined carefully because these alterations suggest malignant transformation into melanoma.

Management: Nevi are excised for biopsy, cosmetic reasons, or repeated inflammation. Nevi that experience recurrent trauma because of their

Clinical features of melanocytic nevi	
Type of melanocytic nevi	**Clinical features**
Congenital	Present at birth; usually greater than 1 cm in diameter; can become prominent and hairy; vary from light brown to black; 5% carry risk of malignancy
Junctional	Flat macules up to 1 cm in size; round or oval; light to dark brown in color; usually found on palms, soles, and genitalia
Intradermal	Dome-shaped papule or nodule; seen on face and neck; may or may not be pigmented
Compound	Macules usually smaller than 1 cm; vary in pigmentation; occur anywhere; larger lesions may develop warty surface
Spitz	Firm, red-brown nodule; usually occur in children on face; growth initially rapid; dermal vessels are dilated
Blue	Usually solitary; blue in color; common on hands and feet
Halo (Sutton's)	Seen on trunk of adolescents and children; indicative of destruction of nevi cells by body's defense system; white halo of pigmentation surrounds existing nevus; there is an association with vitiligo
Becker's	Rare; unilateral lesion in adolescent males; hyperpigmented, becoming hairy; found on back and chest

Fig. 8.10 Clinical features of melanocytic nevi.

site are also excised. Nevi may also be removed prophylactically (e.g., a large, hairy, congenital nevus that has an increased risk of malignant change).

Vascular nevi

Vascular nevi are often present at birth. Most lesions are caused by superficial capillary networks; larger angiomas are caused by deeper, multivascular plexuses.

Port-wine stain: Also known as nevus flammeus, a port-wine stain is a large, irregular, red-purple macule that can affect the face asymmetrically. In later life, it may become darker and nodular.

Salmon patch: As the most common vascular nevus, the salmon patch lesion presents in half of all newborns. The pink patches situated on the upper eyelid often clear rapidly, but those at the back of the neck—"stork-mark" patches—may persist.

Strawberry nevus: Also known as a capillary–cavernous hemangioma, strawberry nevi usually develop soon after birth, growing to a maximum size at 1 year. The nevus begins to involute at 2 years and has usually resolved by the age of 7 years. Strawberry nevi can occur anywhere on the surface of the skin and leave an atrophic area behind after healing.

Cavernous hemangioma: A similar lesion to a strawberry nevi, the cavernous hemangioma lesion presents as a nodule and may not involute completely. The risk of trapped platelets may lead to

thrombocytopenia, and so a course of prednisolone, or even surgery, may be necessary.

Epidermal nevi: These linear epidermal lesions are warty and pigmented, presenting at birth or in early childhood. Epidermal nevi can range from a few centimeters long to a length that covers a whole limb; they may recur after excision. A scalp variant, nevus sebaceous, may become neoplastic and should be removed.

Connective tissue nevi: Presenting as smooth, skin-colored papules or plaques, connective tissue nevi lesions are rare. They may be single or multiple lesions.

Malignant melanoma
Epidemiology

A malignant tumor of melanocytes is known as a melanoma: this is the most lethal of skin tumors. The etiology is unknown, but intensive exposure to ultraviolet light over short periods, such as that experienced while sunbathing, is thought to have a positive correlation with the development of melanomas. There are 10 cases in every 100,000 individuals per year, and the incidence is rising rapidly. The male:female ratio is 1:2, and melanomas can develop in anyone over the age of 20 years. Melanomas tend to develop on areas exposed to the sun: the back is the most common site in men and the leg in women, where half of all cases occur.

Variants of malignant melanoma	
Variant	**Clinical features**
Superficial spreading	Occurs commonly in women; mainly on lower leg; macular; variable pigmentation; can regress
Lentigo	Develops in longstanding lentigo maligna (macular lesion arising in older adults on sun-damaged skin); most common on face
Acral lentiginous	Affects palms, soles, and nail beds; often diagnosed late so has poor survival rates; most common malignant melanoma in mongoloids
Nodular	Occurs commonly in men; usually arises on trunk; pigmented nodule that may rapidly grow and ulcerate

Fig. 8.11 Main variants of malignant melanoma.

Prognosis and tumor depth	
Depth of tumor (mm)	**5-year survival rate (%)**
<1.49	93
1.5–3.49	67
>3.5	38

Fig. 8.12 Prognosis related to tumor depth.

Pathology

Approximately 30% of lesions develop on the site of a preexisting melanocytic nevus; the risk of neoplastic change is greatest in congenital nevi. Individuals with multiple melanocytic nevi (more than 100) or previous malignant melanoma and those with a fair complexion (especially people with red hair and blue eyes) who burn easily in the sun are at increased risk. Local invasion is staged by the Breslow scale, with which the depth of the lesion is measured in millimeters.

Clinical features

The four main variants of malignant melanoma are listed in Fig. 8.11. The prognosis relates to the depth of tumor (Fig. 8.12).

Management

Malignant melanomas are treated by surgical excision. A margin of healthy skin is excised alongside the tumor: 1 cm for tumors less than 1 mm thick, and 3 cm for tumors more than 1 mm thick. Close follow-up is needed to detect recurrence, which may occur locally or through metastases.

Public heath education in the general population will help to detect early malignant changes and prevent excessive future sun exposure.

Malignant epidermal tumors
Basal cell carcinoma
Etiology
Otherwise known as rodent ulcers, basal cell carcinoma is the most common type of skin cancer. The condition arises from basal keratinocytes in the epidermis and most commonly develops in middle-aged to older individuals.

Basal cell carcinoma is most commonly caused by excessive sun exposure, but it can also result from irradiation, chronic scarring, and ingestion of arsenic. There is also some evidence of genetic predisposition. Fair-skinned individuals are most at risk, and the incidence is greater in men than women.

Pathology
The tumor is composed of basophilic cells that bud down from the epidermis to invade the dermis. They may also invade in a lobular fashion (Fig. 8.13).

Clinical features
The lesions tend to arise in sun-exposed areas of the face, such as the nose, eyelids, and temple. They grow slowly and are locally invasive: lesions may have existed for 2 or more years before the patient presents (Plate 15).

Management
If possible, complete excision is the best treatment; this can be difficult if lesions are around the eye or nasolabial fold. Incisional biopsy and radiotherapy

153

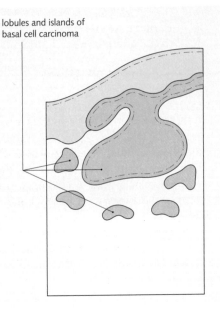

lobules and islands of
basal cell carcinoma

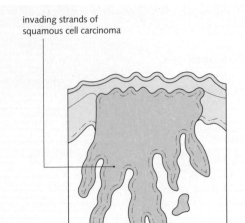

invading strands of
squamous cell carcinoma

Fig. 8.13 Histopathology of basal cell carcinoma (adapted from *Dermatology: An Illustrated Color Text,* 2nd ed., by Gawkrodger DJ, Churchill Livingstone, 1997).

Fig. 8.14 Histopathology of squamous cell carcinoma (adapted from *Dermatology: An Illustrated Color Text,* 2nd ed., by Gawkrodger DJ, Churchill Livingstone, 1997).

may be used in patients who are more than 60 years of age. Cryosurgery may also be used on superficial trunk lesions.

Squamous cell carcinoma
Etiology
Squamous cell carcinoma arises from well-differentiated keratinocytes and usually develops in an area of damaged skin. The risk factors for this condition include:
- Chronic sun exposure, causing actinic damage.
- Irradiation.
- Chronic ulceration/scarring.
- Industrial and tobacco carcinogens.

Other diseases such as viral infections (viral warts) and genetic disorders (xeroderma pigmentosum) may predispose an individual to squamous cell carcinoma. The lesions usually occur in those more than 55 years of age and are more common in men than in women. The tumor may metastasize.

Pathology
The dermoepidermal junction is destroyed by the malignant keratinocytes, which then invade the dermis (Fig. 8.14).

Clinical features
The lesions, which are usually found on sun-exposed sites such as the face, neck, forearm, and hand, begin as small papules that progress to ulcerated, crusted lesions. Squamous cell carcinoma may also present as a dome-shaped nodule (Plate 16). Primary sites of metastatic basal cell carcinoma are usually found around the edges of ulcers, near scars, or in areas of irradiation.

Management
Surgical excision is the first line of management, although tumors of the face and scalp may be treated by incisional biopsy and radiotherapy. Lymph nodes should be examined for metastases.

Other tumors of the skin
Intraepidermal carcinoma (Bowen's disease)
Intraepidermal carcinoma is a form of cancer that is common in older women and presents as either solitary or multiple lesions. The trunk and lower legs are mainly affected, with lightly pigmented scaly lesions reaching several centimeters in size. Histologically, there are atypical but nonkeratinized keratinocytes present, and a thickening of the epidermis occurs. Arsenic exposure is a major risk factor, and conversion to squamous cell carcinoma

may rarely occur. Treatment is by excision, curettage, or cryotherapy.

Keratoacanthoma

A keratoacanthoma is a nonmalignant, rapidly growing tumor that arises in sun-exposed areas. It forms a dome-shaped papule complete with a central keratin plug, which may leave a crater if removed. The lesion resembles a squamous cell carcinoma histologically; however, the lesion is differentiated from this carcinoma by a more symmetrical pattern. The lesion will resolve spontaneously within a few months but leaves scarring; removal of the keratoacanthoma is preferable.

Cutaneous T cell lymphoma

Also known as mycosis fungoides, a cutaneous T cell lymphoma results from a lymphoma that develops in normal skin tissue. The tumor grows slowly and may lead to secondary skin deposits. The four stages of development are as follows:

- Premycotic plaques—these are similar to those present in psoriasis.
- Infiltrated plaques—fixed plaques develop, most commonly on the trunk.
- Tumor stage—within the plaques, nodules and ulcers develop.
- Systemic disease—the tumor spreads to lymph nodes and organs.

Treatment is aimed at containing the lymphoma—topical steroids can be used to control the premycotic plaques. UVB therapy, PUVA therapy, topical nitrogen mustard application, photopheresis, radiotherapy, and chemotherapy are also possible treatments that have varying degrees of effect.

Kaposi's sarcoma

Kaposi's sarcoma is a neoplasm characterised by multifocal vascular skin tumors seen in around 33% of patients with AIDS. Arising from vascular endothelium and presenting as purple or dark brown nodules or plaque on the face, mouth, limbs, or trunk, it may also invade internal organs. This sarcoma may result from infection with herpesvirus 8. A variation of Kaposi's sarcoma, seen in older Jewish men from Eastern Europe, is more benign and is not associated with HIV. Treatment includes radiotherapy and X-ray therapy. Because the clinical course is dominated by infections, treatment does not help prolong the life of most patients.

Disorders of specific skin structures

Sweat and sebaceous glands

Acne vulgaris

Pathology

Acne is one of the most common diseases of skin. Its various lesions (comedones, papules, pustules, cysts, and scars) result from chronic inflammation of the pilosebaceous apparatus; acne vulgaris affects mainly the face, shoulders, and trunk. It commonly presents around puberty and appears in women earlier than men, although both sexes are affected equally. Acne is essentially caused by excessive production of sebum, hyperkeratosis of the pilosebaceous duct, and colonization with *Propionibacterium acnes*. These lead to a release of inflammatory cytokines that results in inflammation.

Clinical features

There are five main lesions in acne: comedones, papules, pustules, cysts, and scars.

Comedones: Comedones are classified as either open or closed. Open comedones are dilated pores with a plug of keratin that contains melanin (blackheads). Closed comedones are small, cream-colored papules (whiteheads).

Other lesions: Comedones progress to inflammatory papules, pustules, and cysts found on sites that have a preponderance of sebaceous glands: the face, shoulders, back, and upper chest (Plate 17). Cysts are the most destructive of the lesions in acne: upon healing, they leave scars that may be "ice-pick," keloidal, or atrophic.

Complications

Although acne itself is a relatively harmless disease, the psychological effects it has on young patients should not be underestimated. Patients severely devalue their own self-image because of the disorder and, consequently, suffer shame and lack of self-confidence. Upon successful physical treatment of acne, the psychological symptoms often improve.

Management

Fig. 8.15 lists a variety of treatments for acne.

Rosacea

Rosacea is an erythematous, pustular dermatitis that affects the face. The etiology is unknown; histology

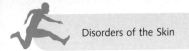
Treatment of acne vulgaris	
Treatment	**Comments**
Benzoyl peroxide cream	Eradicates *P. acnes*; bleaches clothes, may cause irritation and contact allergies
Tretinoin	Treats comedones before they evolve, but may cause irritation
Antibiotics	First-line: tetracycline; second-line: erythromycin and trimethoprim; antibiotics are suppressive, not curative; they are thought to affect lipase-producing bacteria present in pilosebaceous follicles
Antiandrogens	Used in combination with an estrogen in women only; anti-androgens suppress sebum production
Retinoid	Isotretinoin reduces sebum production, inhibits *P. acnes*, and is anti-inflammatory; women must not be pregnant and must take oral contraceptive pill throughout 6-month course becauase retinoids are teratogenic; side effects can be severe
Triamcinolone acetonide	Steroid injected into acne cyst to aid healing
Non-drug therapies	Excision, cryotherapy, removal of comedones using an extractor

Fig. 8.15 Treatment of acne vulgaris.

shows dilated dermal blood vessels, sebaceous gland enlargement, and inflammatory cell changes.

Clinical features

The first sign of rosacea is facial flushing. This is followed by the development of erythema, telangiectasia, papules, and pustules (Plate 18). It occurs most commonly in middle-aged individuals although all age groups can be affected.

Complications

Complications include lymphedema of the face, hypertrophy of the connective tissue and sebaceous glands of the nose (rhinophyma-hyperplasia), and blepharitis and conjunctivitis.

Management

Metronidazole gel is used twice a day; if the rosacea proves resistant, oral tetracycline is started. Isotretinoin can also be used. Surgical correction is required for rhinophyma-hyperplasia.

Other disorders
Perioral dermatitis

A side effect of topical steroids, perioral dermatitis presents as papules and pustules around the mouth and chin. It is treated effectively with oral tetracycline.

Hydradenitis suppurativa

Hydradenitis suppurativa describes the chronic inflammation of the apocrine sweat glands. Nodules, abscesses, cysts, and sinuses develop in the axillae,

groin and perineum, and may result in permanent scarring. Treatment depends on the severity of the condition and includes topical antiseptics, systemic antibiotics, and excision.

Hyperhidrosis

Hyperhidrosis is excessive sweating caused by eccrine gland overactivity. It usually arises from heightened emotion, but hypoglycemia and shock may also stimulate the sweat glands. The condition can be managed by the application of 20% aluminum chloride in alcohol.

Hair disorders
Alopecia
Classification

Diffuse nonscarring: In individuals with diffuse nonscarring, diffuse hair loss occurs across the whole scalp. It may be androgen-dependent (common male pattern baldness, Fig. 8.16), meaning the follicles are slowly converted from terminal to vellus hairs, and is present in 80% of men by the age of 70 years. Androgenic alopecia also occurs in postmenopausal women to a lesser extent.

Diffuse nonscarring alopecia is also caused by endocrine disorders: underactivity of the thyroid, pituitary, and adrenal glands can all cause alopecia, as can a dietary protein, iron, or zinc deficiency. Telogen effluvium can result in diffuse nonscarring alopecia, as can the ingestion of certain drugs such as heparin and warfarin.

Localized nonscarring: Patchy hair loss may be caused by infection (tinea capitis), trauma, or alopecia areata. This condition can cause patchy baldness or complete hair loss and is associated with autoimmune disorders. It is characterized by pathognomonic "exclamation mark" hairs—dystrophic, depigmented hairs that are short and taper toward the margins of hair loss. The hair loss appears to be caused by the anagen stage being prematurely arrested and begins at 20–30 years of age. If the alopecia areata is localized, regrowth may occur, but the course of the disorder is unpredictable. It can be treated to some extent by triamcinolone acetonide and PUVA.

Scarring (cicatricial) alopecia: Scarring results from the destruction of hair follicles. The destruction can be caused by burns, irradiation, infection (e.g., shingles, kerion, or tertiary syphilis), lichen planus, lupus erythematosus, and pseudopelade—a term used to describe the end-stage of a destructive inflammatory process of unknown etiology in the scalp.

Excess hair
Hirsutism
The excessive growth of male pattern hair in a female is known as hirsutism. It can be idiopathic, presenting with terminal hair development in the beard area and around the nipples, or, more frequently, it can be drug-induced. Other causes of hirsutism are listed in Fig. 8.17.

Hypertrichosis
The excessive growth of terminal hairs in a nonandrogenic distribution is referred to as hypertrichosis. The condition can be classified into localized (caused by melanocytic nevi, chronic scarring, and inflammation) or generalized (caused by anorexia nervosa, malnutrition, underlying malignancy, and drugs). Investigation is important in finding the underlying cause.

Other disorders
Hair shaft defects
Usually genetic in origin, hair shaft defects are rare but can result in brittle, beaded, and broken hair shafts.

Dandruff
The normal scalp is layered with fine scales of keratin; dandruff is simply a physiologic exaggeration

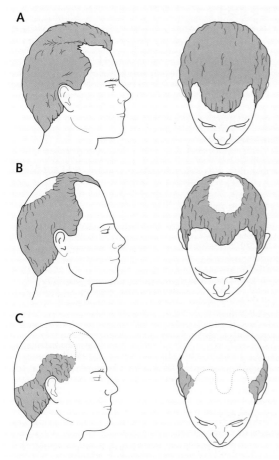

Fig. 8.16 Male pattern baldness. A. Bitemporal recession. B. Vertex involvement. C. Most severe pattern of male baldness (adapted with permission from *Dermatology: An Illustrated Color Text*, 2nd ed., by Gawkrodger DJ, Churchill Livingstone, 1997).

Other causes of hirsutism	
Cause of hirsutism	**Example of disease**
Endocrine	Acromegaly
	Cushing's syndrome
	Virilizing tumors
	Congenital adrenal hyperplasia
Ovarian	Polycystic ovaries
Iatrogenic	Excess androgens
	Excess progesterones
Idiopathic	End-organ hypersensitivity to androgen

Fig. 8.17 Other causes of hirsutism.

157

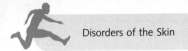
of the normal exfoliative process. Certain conditions (e.g., seborrheic dermatitis of the scalp and psoriasis) can produce severe scaling of the scalp that may be mistaken for dandruff.

Tinea capitis

Tinea capitis is ringworm of the scalp that may cause alopecia.

Nail disorders
Congenital disease
Nail-patella syndrome

Inherited in a Mendelian-dominant fashion, nail-patella syndrome is a disorder in which the nails and the patella are rudimentary or absent. The thumb is always affected; other digits may or may not be spared.

Paronychia congenita

An individual's nails are thickened and discolored in this autosomal dominant disorder termed paronychia congenita; the individual may also experience palmar-plantar keratoderma, with or without hyperhidrosis. There is a risk of malignant mucosal dysplasia.

Trauma
Subungual hematoma

Subungual hematomas are traumatic lesions that occur when the nail has undergone increased pressure (e.g., fingernail trapped in the door; toenail stood on). The possibility of a malignant cause, however, must always be considered with this condition.

Splinter hemorrhages

Although commonly due to trauma, splinter hemorrhages may also indicate infective endocarditis.

Ingrown toenails

Two factors contribute to ingrown toenails: ill-fitting shoes predispose a person to deformities of the feet, and, if the wrong method of cutting toenails is employed, spicules of nail are left that damage the nail fold. The nail of the big toe is most often involved, and intense discomfort is experienced.

Onychogryphosis

Chronic trauma predisposes an individual to onychogryphosis, a condition in which the hallux toenails become grossly thickened and horn-like.

Brittle nails

Brittle nails are usually caused by heavy exposure to detergents and water, and patients often present with this condition as a common complaint. This condition may also be caused by iron deficiency, hypothyroidism, and digital ischemia.

Nail involvement in the dermatoses
Psoriasis

Psoriatic nail involvement causes pitting, nail thickening, onycholysis, discoloration, and subungual hyperkeratosis.

Alopecia areata

Fine pitting and rough nail surfaces are features of alopecia areata.

Eczema

Nail features of eczema include coarse pitting, transverse ridging, dystrophy, and shiny nails caused by rubbing.

Lichen planus

Lichen planus leads to a thinned nail plate, longitudinal grooves, adhesions between the nail fold and the nail bed, and loss of the nail.

Infections
Tinea unguium

A tinea unguium fungal infection spreads to the free edge of the nail and spreads distally to involve the whole nail. As a result, the nail becomes thickened, yellow, and crumbly and subungual hyperkeratosis can be seen (Plate 19). Toenails are involved more than fingernails, but very rarely are all the nails on one hand and foot involved. Treatment is with topical or oral imidazoles such as clotrimazole and ketoconazole. Systemic treatment with Griseofulvin is employed in more severe infections.

Chronic paronychia (Candida albicans)

A condition called chronic paronychia is often seen in individuals who work in wet environments. The nail becomes boggy, the cuticle is detached, and pressure on the nail will cause pus to be extruded. Secondary involvement of the nail matrix can result in an abnormally ridged nail, and the nail plate may become infected.

Management involves avoiding wet work by wearing rubber gloves and taking simple antiseptics and applying clotrimazole or amphotericin B lotion. Cauterization of the subcuticular space may be necessary in resistant cases: this treatment is performed by inserting a cotton wick soaked in phenol into the space for 1 minute.

Acute bacterial paronychia
Originating at the junction of the posterior and lateral folds, this infection leads to pus formation. Management includes hot compresses, drainage, and a systemic antibiotic, such as oral floxacillin.

Tumors of the nails
Viral warts
Periungual warts often occur; treatment is the same as for warts located elsewhere on the body.

Periungual fibromas
Periungual fibromas are a complication of tuberous sclerosis and appear during puberty.

Myxoid cysts
Mucous cysts called myxoid cysts are found adjacent to the proximal fingernail fold; they contain clear fluid and are fluctuant. They can be treated with cryotherapy, steroid injection, or excision.

Malignant melanoma
If a pigmented streak appears in the nail, a biopsy must be performed to exclude a malignant melanoma. Biopsies must also be performed on all atypical or ulcerating lesions around the nail fold.

Nail changes in systemic disease
Nails often show nonspecific changes in systemic disease, the most important of which is clubbing. Discoloration, koilonychia, onycholysis, pitting, and ridging are also important signs of systemic disease (Fig. 8.18).

Vascular and lymphatic disorders
Disorders of cutaneous blood vessels
Definitions
Erythema: Redness of the skin caused by vasodilatation is referred to as erythema. It may be localized or generalized.

Flushing: Sudden onset of erythema owing to vasodilatation is called flushing. It is caused by a number of factors, including emotion (blushing), menopause, foods, drugs, rosacea, carcinoid syndrome, and pheochromocytoma.

Telangiectasia: Visible dilatation of dermal venules or arterioles (spider nevi) is termed telangiectasia. This condition can result from skin atrophy, excessive estrogen, connective tissue disease, rosacea, or venous disease—or it may be congenital. The lesions can be treated with needle cautery (electrodessication) and lasers.

Purpura: A discoloration of the skin caused by the extravasation of blood cells refers to purpura, which may be caused by a number of factors: vessel wall

Nail changes in systemic disease	
Nail change	**Causes**
Beau's lines (transverse grooves)	Severe systemic illness
Brittle nails	Iron deficiency, hypothryoidism, loss of blood supply to nails, exposure to water and chemicals
Color change	Drugs, cyanosis, infection, trauma, renal failure, nicotine staining, psoriasis
Clubbing	Bronchial carcinoma, fibrosing alveolitis, asbestosis, infective endocarditis, congenital cyanotic defects, inflammatory bowel disease, thyrotoxicosis, biliary cirrhosis
Koilonychia (spoon-shaped nail)	Iron deficiency anemia, lichen planus, chemical exposure
Nail fold telangiectasia (dilated capillaries)	Connective tissue disorders
Onycholysis (separation of nail from bed)	Psoriasis, fungal infection, trauma, thyrotoxicosis, drugs (tetracyclines)
Pitting	Psoriasis, eczema, alopecia, lichen planus
Ridging (transverse and longitudinal)	Eczema, psoriasis, lichen planus

Fig. 8.18 Nail changes in systemic disease.

defects, defective dermal support, clotting defects, or idiopathic pigmented purpura.

Raynaud's phenomenon

Raynaud's phenomenon is a three-stage process caused by paroxysmal vasoconstriction and affects mainly women. The fingers first turn white due to ischemia, and then they turn blue due to cyanosis caused by pooled, deoxygenated blood in capillaries. Finally, the fingers turn red due to reactive hyperemia as the capillaries perfuse again. Causes of Raynaud's phenomenon include:

- Arterial occlusion.
- Connective tissue disease.
- Hyperviscosity of blood.
- Neurologic defects.
- Vasoconstriction caused by use of vibrating tools.
- Toxins and drugs.

Because the phenomenon is often precipitated by cold, affected patients are advised to keep their hands warm. Taking prazosin and phenoxybenzamine may also help.

Livedo reticularis

Cyanosis occurring in a marble pattern on the skin is called livedo reticularis. It is caused by reduced arteriole flow and poor skin circulation; reversible livedo is usually induced by cold and is seen in children, while fixed livedo is usually caused by vasculitis and requires further investigation.

Chilblains

Chilblains are painful, purple-pink inflamed swellings found on the fingers, toes, and ears and are cold to the touch. The lesions may last for weeks and may be complicated by ulceration. Chilblains are much less common since the introduction of central heating.

Lymphatic disorders and the skin
Lymphedema

Secondary lymphedema is caused by inadequate lymphatic drainage, which may be due to:

- Recurrent infection.
- Blockage.
- Surgical or irradiation destruction.

Primary lymphedema may follow infection and usually presents in adolescence. Lymphedematous areas are at increased risk of infection, and taking prophylaxis with penicillin may be necessary.

Lymphangitis

Presenting as a tender red line extending from a focus of infection, lymphangitis describes lymphatic vessel infection. It is treated with intravenous antibiotics.

Leg ulcers
Etiology

Leg ulcers can be caused by venous disease, arterial disease, vasculitic disease, or neuropathy (Fig. 8.19). They affect 1% of the adult population and are twice as common in women as in men.

Pathology

Venous ulcers: Valve incompetence in perforating veins leads to increased capillary hydrostatic pressure and permeability. Fibrin deposits form adjacent to the capillaries and interfere with nutrient exchange, leading to ulceration. Usually presenting in middle age to later life, risk factors for development of venous ulcers include obesity and venous thrombosis. The first signs are a feeling of heaviness in the legs caused by edema; discoloration of the skin and eczema may subsequently occur. Fibrosis of the dermis and subcutis (lipodermatosclerosis) leads to ulceration, which often follows minor trauma. The ulcer usually affects the medial and sometimes the lateral malleolus (Plate 20). Ulcers are exudative to begin with but may then enter a granulomatous healing phase, which lasts for months.

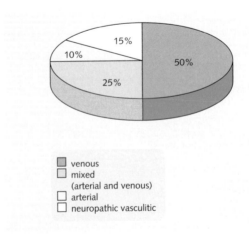

venous
mixed
(arterial and venous)
arterial
neuropathic vasculitic

Fig. 8.19 Percentages of leg ulcers caused by venous disease, arterial disease, vasculitis disease, or neuropathy.

Some larger venous ulcers may never heal. The post-ulcer leg has a slender, sclerosed ankle caused by fibrosis.

Arterial ulcers: Arterial disease leads to ischemia, with reduced circulation and consequently reduced temperature in the leg; hair loss, toenail dystrophy, and cyanosis also occur. Leg ulcers form on the foot or mid-shin and are sharply defined; surrounding pulses are reduced or absent.

Vasculitic ulcers: Vasculitic ulcers begin as a purpuric patch that then becomes necrotic and leads to punched-out lesions.

Neuropathic ulcers: Neuropathic ulcers occur on the foot and are a result of neurologic disease, including diabetic polyneuropathy.

Complications

Neglected ulcers may enlarge and become difficult to manage. Specific complications of venous ulcers include infection, lymphedema, contact dermatitis (sensitivity to topical treatment), and, rarely, malignant change to squamous cell carcinoma.

Management

Treatment of underlying factors—obesity, cardiac failure, anemia, and arthritis—is helpful; other treatments include:

- Compression bandages to increase venous return and reduce edema—this treatment is contraindicated in arterial ulcers, so Doppler studies must be carried out to exclude coexisting arterial disease before treatment is initiated.
- Elevation, exercise, and diet to encourage normal blood flow.
- Topical therapy—antiseptics, desloughing agents, colloid or gel dressings, low-adherent bandages, medicated dressings, and other such treatments are common practice.
- Oral therapy—analgesia is the main type of therapy, but diuretics and antibiotics are used to treat secondary infection.
- Reconstructive vein surgery—this procedure is only helpful in younger patients.

Vasculitis and reactive erythema
Vasculitis

Inflammation of small- to medium-sized blood vessels is referred to as vasculitis. This condition is commonly caused by circulating immune complexes that lodge in the vessel walls and activate complement, causing damage to the vessel walls. The disease is usually detected through characteristic skin changes, such as palpable purpura over the legs and buttocks that are often painful. Vasculitis may affect only the skin, or it may also spread to the joints, kidneys, lungs, gut, and nervous system (Fig. 8.20). Cutaneous vasculitis is treated successfully with dapsone and oral steroids.

Erythema multiforme

Erythema multiforme is an immune-mediated disease characterized by target lesions consisting of red rings with a pale central area that may blister.

Types of vasculitis	
	Clinical features
Henoch-Schönlein purpura	Cutaneous signs accompanied by arthritis, abdominal pain and hematuria; it often follows a streptococcal infection and mainly affects children
Nodular vasculitis	Painful subcutaneous nodules are found on the lower legs
Polyarteritis nodosa	An uncommon necrotizing vasculitis that affects middle-aged men; subcutaneous nodules develop, together with hypertension, renal failure, and neuropathy
Wegener's granulomatosis	A rare and potentially fatal vasculitis; malaise, lung involvement, and glomerulonephritis are accompanied by cutaneous vasculitis in 50% of patients
Giant cell arteritis	Affects older adults who present with scalp tenderness owing to temporal artery involvement, which can cause scalp necrosis; prednisolone should be given, or sight may be lost

Fig. 8.20 Types of vasculitis.

161

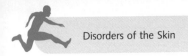
Mucosa may be involved. The disease is caused by circulating immune complexes that are deposited in blood vessel walls; histologic features include a necrotic epidermis, edema in the dermis, an inflammatory infiltrate, and vasodilatation. Underlying causes include viral, bacterial, and fungal infections; drugs; pregnancy; and malignancy. Management is by treatment of the underlying cause and systemic steroids to modify the acute symptoms.

Erythema nodosum

Erythema nodosum is an inflammation of subcutaneous fat and causes painful red-blue nodules on the calves and shins. The female:male ratio is 3:1. Circulating immune complexes play an important role in the pathology, and the causes of erythema nodosum include infection, drugs, inflammatory bowel disease, and sarcoidosis. Joint pain and fever often accompany the nodules, and the disease usually clears spontaneously after 2 months, so treatment is rarely needed.

Sweet's disease

Sweet's disease is an acute, febrile, neutrophilic dermatosis that is characterized by red, annular plaques on the face and limbs. The lesions are accompanied by fever and a raised neutrophil count. Treatment with prednisolone is usually effective.

Graft-versus-host disease

The condition of donor lymphocytes reacting against host tissue is known as graft-versus-host disease. This disease usually affects patients who have undergone a bone marrow transplant and causes fever, malaise, and an acute eruption that may progress to toxic epidermal necrolysis. A skin biopsy helps with the diagnosis, and systemic steroids are usually necessary in management.

Disorders of pigmentation

Hypopigmentation
Vitiligo
Etiology

Vitiligo is a common acquired idiopathic disorder that leads to patchy, scaled macules (Plate 21). There is an association with pernicious anemia, thyroid disease, and Addison's disease, with about 30% of patients having a positive family history. The onset is usually between 10 and 30 years of age; the male:

female ratio is 1:1, and it affects around 0.5% of the population.

Clinical features

Vitiligo may be precipitated by trauma or sunburn. The well-defined white macules are usually symmetrical and frequently affect the hands, wrists, knees, neck, and areas surrounding orifices.

Complications

Because melanocytes are absent from lesions, care must be taken when skin is exposed to the sun.

Management

Camouflage cosmetics often prove unsatisfactory. Sunscreen helps to reduce the contrast between tanned skin and patches of vitiligo, and, in darker skin, topical steroids may induce repigmentation. When vitiligo is nearly universal and very noticeable, induced depigmentation of remaining normal skin can be caused by 20% hydroquinone ointment.

Albinism

Albinism is an autosomal recessive disorder that has a prevalence of 1 in 20,000. In this condition, melanocytes fail to synthesize melanin, leading to a lack of pigment in the skin. In addition to the skin being pale, the hair is white, and the eyes lack pigmentation. Patients suffer from photophobia, nystagmus, and poor sight. Because the body has no protection against ultraviolet rays, the sun should be strictly avoided; the risk of squamous cell carcinoma is greatly increased.

Phenylketonuria

Phenylketonuria is an autosomal recessive metabolic defect. The enzyme that converts phenylalanine into tyrosine is missing, which leads to the accumulation of metabolites in the brain. If left untreated, mental retardation and choreoathetosis may occur. The hair and skin are fair because melanin synthesis is impaired. In addition, atopic eczema is common. Treatment is through a diet low in phenylalanine.

Hyperpigmentation
Freckles and lentigines

Freckles are small, light brown macules that develop in sun-exposed areas of the skin. Freckles darken upon intense ultraviolet exposure: they have normal numbers of melanocytes, but, upon stimulation, synthesis of melanin is increased. They are common and are frequently seen on many faces over the summer months. Lentigines are dark brown macules that do not darken in the sun; they have an increased number of melanocytes. Lentigines may respond to cryotherapy.

Chloasma
Induced by pregnancy or by taking the oral contraception pill, chloasma is a symmetrical facial pigmentation that often involves the forehead. It improves spontaneously, although sunscreens and camouflage cosmetics may help.

Drug-induced pigmentation
Pigmentation is a common effect of some drugs, such as phenothiazine, minocycline, amiodarone, clofazimine, chlorpromazine, and antimalarials.

Other causes
Peutz-Jeghers syndrome causes lentigines to form around the lips, mucosa, and fingers; these lesions are associated with the small bowel polyps of the disease. Addison's disease leads to melanogenesis through the production of excess adrenocorticotrophic hormone; pigmentation occurs on buccal mucosa, palmar creases, scars, and flexures.

Blistering disorders

Pemphigus
Pathology
Pemphigus is a potentially fatal disease that affects both sexes equally and usually presents in middle-aged or older individuals, with the mean age of onset being around the sixth decade. About 90% of patients have circulating IgG autoantibodies that bind to the skin's intracellular matrix, inducing the release of proteolytic enzymes from adjacent keratinocytes. This subsequently causes intraepidermal splits, resulting in thin-walled, fragile blisters. Pemphigus also has an association with other autoimmune disorders.

Clinical features
The disease presents in one-half of patients as an eruption of shallow blisters around the mouth; further lesions follow several months later on the face and trunk of all affected individuals. Blisters invariably rupture, so the disease tends to present with skin erosions more predominant than blisters. This is in contrast to pemphigoid, which is characterized by thicker and more robust blister walls.

Management
Systemic steroids, usually oral prednisolone, are given in high doses to control the blistering and are often administered in tandem with an immunosuppressive drug such as azathioprine. The steroids are continued at a lower dose for years; at this stage, the mortality and morbidity from steroid side effects and immunosuppression are equal to that of the disease itself.

Pemphigoid
Pathology
Affecting older adults, pemphigoid is characterized by a chronic blistering eruption. The pathology is similar to that of pemphigus, with the exception that IgG antibodies are deposited at the basement membrane. Circulating IgG antibodies are present in 70% of patients. The damage is deeper than in pemphigus; therefore, the blisters have a thicker wall and are less likely to rupture.

Clinical features
Pemphigoid has three different patterns as shown in Fig. 8.21.

	Clinical patterns of pemphigoid
Type of pemphigoid	**Clinical features**
Bullous	Large, tense blisters that usually affect older adults; trunk, limbs, and flexures are affected; 10% of patients have oral lesions; may be preceded by urticaria; may be localized to a single site (Plate 22)
Cicatricial	Ocular and oral mucosa affected; post-pemphigoid scarring may affect sight
Pemphigoid (herpes) gestationis	Bullous lesions that are associated with pregnancy; clears after delivery but may recur in subsequent pregnancies

Fig. 8.21 Clinical patterns of pemphigoid.

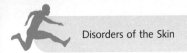
Management

Oral prednisolone is prescribed at a lower dose than for pemphigus; the disease is self-limiting in half of all cases; in the other half, steroids can be stopped after 2 years. Azathioprine may also be prescribed.

Dermatitis herpetiformis

Pathology

Dermatitis herpetiformis features a symmetrical eruption of pruritic blisters and usually presents in the third or fourth decade of life. IgA can be seen at the dermal papillae when viewed through immunofluorescence; jejunal villus atrophy is also present in the majority of cases. The clinical signs respond well to a gluten-free diet, suggesting that gluten sensitivity is present in both the gut and the skin. The male:female ratio is 2:1.

Clinical features

The first sign of dermatitis herpetiformis is usually a group of small, itchy vesicles that erupt on the scalp, elbows, knees, and buttocks. Although small bowel pathology is often present, gastrointestinal symptoms are uncommon.

Inherited disorders of the skin

The ichthyoses

The ichthyoses are a group of disorders characterized by dry and scaly skin. The inheritance is autosomal dominant, with the exception of X-linked ichthyosis. The different types of ichthyoses are listed in Fig. 8.22.

Management

Regular use of emollients and moisturizing creams are the mainstays of treatment. Neonatal ichthyoses must be managed in a pediatric intensive care unit because thermoregulation is disturbed and fluid losses may be significant.

Keratoderma

Keratoderma is characterized by gross hyperkeratosis of the palms and soles. The disorder can also be acquired or inherited. Tylosis (callus formation) describes the typical diffuse pattern of hyperkeratosis; in some patients, the disorder is associated with esophageal carcinoma. Keratoma is treated with keratolytics, such as salicylic acid ointment or urea cream.

Epidermolysis bullosa

Minor injury or trauma induces blistering in patients with epidermolysis bullosa. The disease ranges in severity from simple epidermolysis bullosa (the most common type, which features blisters limited to areas affected by friction) to junctional epidermolysis bullosa, a rare and potentially fatal disorder

Classification of ichthyoses			
Type of ichthyosis	Mode of inheritance	Incidence	Clinical features
Ichthyosis vulgaris	Autosomal dominant	1:250 births	Disorder of epidermal cornification; onset between 1 and 4 years; granular layer is reduced or absent; dry skin with white scales on back and extensor surface of limbs; palmar and plantar markings are increased
X-linked ichthyosis	X-linked	1:7000 births	Onset is early; scales are dark and widespread, with face, neck, and scalp all involved; caused by deficiency of steroid sulfatase
Bullous ichthyosiform erythroderma/ epidermolytic hyperkeratosis	Autosomal dominant	1:100,000	Presents at birth; skin is red, moist, and eroded in parts; erythema eventually replaced by scales; flexures particularly affected; hyperkeratosis develops in childhood
Nonbullous ichthyosiform erythroderma	Autosomal dominant	1:100,000	Presents at birth; collodion baby (newborn with tight, shiny skin causing feeding difficulties and ectropion); progresses to reddening and thickening of skin with fine, white scales; acanthosis is present

Fig. 8.22 Classification of ichthyoses.

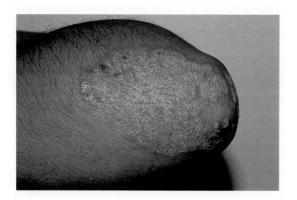

Plate 1 Plaque psoriasis.

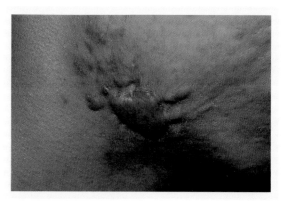

Plate 2 The Koebner phenomenon.

Plate 3 Atopic/flexural eczema.

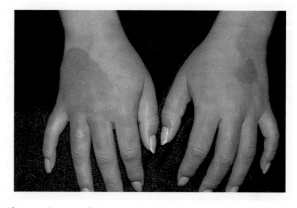

Plate 4 Contact dermatitis.

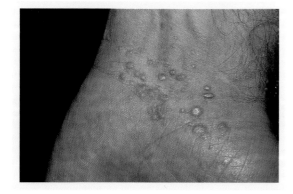

Plate 5 Lichen planus

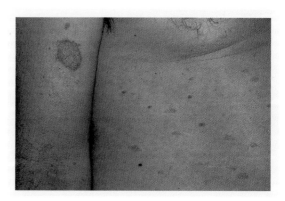

Plate 6 Pityriasis rosea.

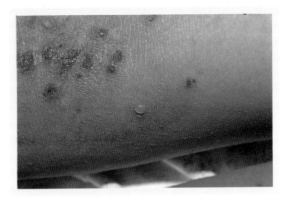

Plate 7 Impetigo.

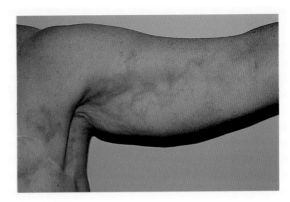

Plate 8 Cellulitis.

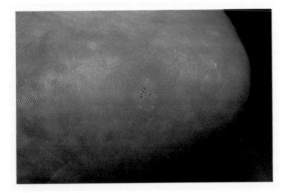

Plate 9 Simple viral wart.

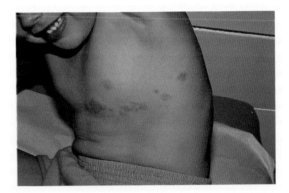

Plate 10 Herpes zoster.

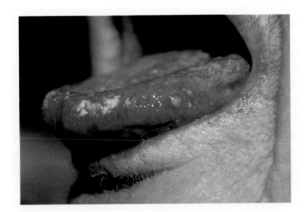

Plate 11 Candida albicans.

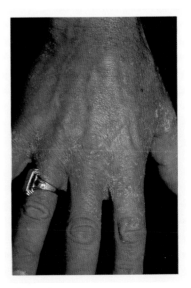

Plate 12 Scabies infestation.

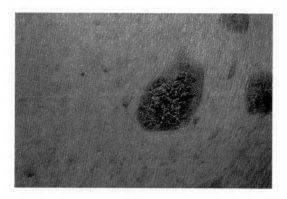

Plate 13 Seborrheic warts.

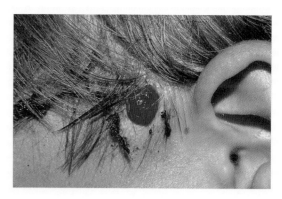

Plate 14 Pyodermic granuloma.

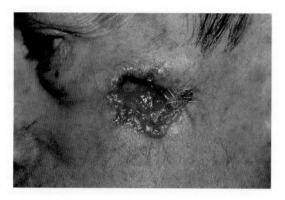

Plate 15 Basal cell carcinoma.

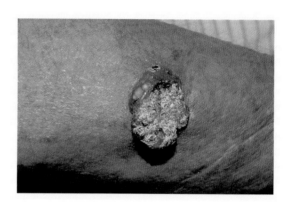

Plate 16 Squamous cell carcinoma.

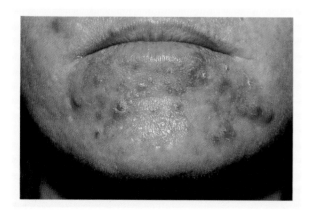

Plate 17 Papulopustular acne.

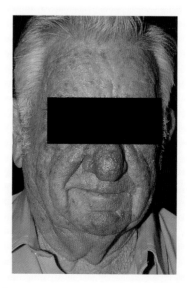

Plate 18 Rosacea.

III

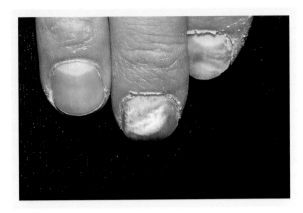

Plate 19 Fungal infection of the nails.

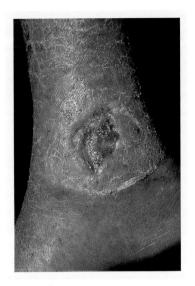

Plate 20 Venous ulcer.

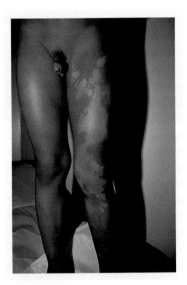

Plate 21 Vitiligo.

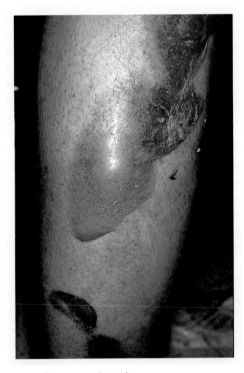

Plate 22 Bulbous pemphigoid.

characterized by large blisters around the bodily orifices at birth. Dystrophic epidermolysis bullosa, which can be inherited in either an autosomal recessive or autosomal dominant manner, causes severe blistering and deformity of the nails. In the recessive form, esophageal stricture and fusion of fingers and toes may occur. The disease is managed in specialized centers, and management relies on the avoidance of trauma and secondary infection.

Neurofibromatosis

Two forms of neurofibromatosis (NF) are recognized: NF1 (von Recklinghausen's peripheral neurofibromatosis) and NF2 (bilateral acoustic central neurofibromatosis). The disease is inherited in an autosomal dominant fashion and affects 1 in 3000 births. Skin involvement includes:

- *Café-au-lait* spots—light brown macules that appear in childhood; six or more macules larger than 2.5 cm in diameter are diagnostic.
- Axillary freckling.
- Cutaneous neurofibromata—smooth sessile nodules that may become pedunculated; gross cutaneous nodular overgrowth leads to elephantiasis neuromatosa.
- Lisch nodules—pigmented hamartomas in the iris.
- Oral lesions.

In 10% of patients, IQ is 70 or less. In 6% of patients, the development of malignant sarcomas is a serious complication. Genetic counseling is an important part of management for patients; excision of nodules may also be appropriate.

Tuberous sclerosis

Tuberous sclerosis is a rare disorder passed on in an autosomal dominant manner, and it is characterized by hamartomas in organs and bone. The cutaneous features include:

- Ash-leaf patches—present in infancy; these are ovoid or elongated hypopigmented macules that fluoresce under a Wood's light.
- Adenoma sebaceum—an acne-like eruption of fibromatous papules around the nose in late childhood and adolescence.
- Periungual fibromata—fibrous pink projections that are visible under the nail folds.
- Shagreen patch—angiofibromatous plaque located on the lower back.

Management involves genetic counseling, attending support groups, and cauterization of the adenoma sebaceum.

Xeroderma pigmentosum

Caused by defective repair of ultraviolet-damaged DNA, xeroderma pigmentosum is characterized by photosensitivity that begins in infancy. The persistent ultraviolet-damaged skin results in the development of skin tumors, which may cause death by 30 years. Affected patients must avoid sunlight. The condition is rare and is autosomal recessive in inheritance.

Pseudoxanthoma elasticum

Pseudoxanthoma elasticum describes a group of four disorders caused by abnormalities in elastin and collagen. It is characterized by loose, wrinkled skin that contains papules and is most often found in the flexures of the neck. The disorders are inherited in both an autosomal dominant and recessive pattern.

Connective tissue disorders in the skin

Lupus erythematosus
Etiology

Approximately 90% of patients with systemic lupus erythematosus (SLE) have circulating antinuclear antibodies detectable in their serum; antibodies to nucleolar and cytoplasmic antigens are also present. SLE is associated with HLA B8 and DR3; patients may also have T suppressor cell dysfunction. In discoid lupus erythematosus (DLE), however, only 25% of patients have circulating antinuclear antibodies.

Pathology

The lesions of DLE are annular lesions with an erythematous margin; these lesions show epidermal atrophy, hyperkeratosis, and basal layer degeneration. SLE shows similar lesions accompanied by dermal edema, inflammation, and, occasionally, vasculitis. Immunoglobulins and complement are deposited at the junction of the epidermis and dermis in the lesions (and in sun-exposed skin in SLE); they can be viewed by direct immunofluorescence.

165

Clinical features

Skin involvement, which is also present in 75% of patients with SLE, includes:

- Erythematous butterfly rash present on the face.
- Photosensitivity.
- Discoid lesions.
- Diffuse alopecia.

To diagnose SLE, other systemic features listed in Fig. 8.23 must also be present.

Clinical features of DLE include discoid lesions that appear on the face, scalp, or hands. The lesions have a well-defined margin and are red, atrophic, and scaly. Follicular keratin plugs may be seen.

Complications

In addition to the systemic features listed in Fig. 8.23, posthealing scarring may lead to alopecia and hypopigmentation in pigmented skin.

Management

DLE can be treated with potent topical steroids; systemic therapy involves administration of chloroquine or immunosuppressive agents. Regular ophthalmic checks are also necessary to detect retinal involvement. Sunscreen is used to protect photosensitive skin.

Systemic sclerosis

Systemic sclerosis is a multisystem disorder that affects the skin in the following ways:

- Raynaud's phenomenon.
- Resorption of finger pulps.
- Tight, waxy, and stiff skin on the fingers, forearms, and calves.
- Perioral furrowing.
- Telangiectasia.

Systemic features, such as renal involvement, may cause death. Treatment is based mainly on education and support, although nifedipine may aid Raynaud's phenomenon.

Localized scleroderma (morphea)

Localized scleroderma is of unknown etiology and causes tight bands of sclerosis on the skin that are accompanied by indurated plaques. The lesions, which affect the trunk and limbs, eventually become pale and shiny, leading to hairless and atrophic areas of skin. The disease resolves spontaneously within a few months.

Dermatomyositis

The skin changes in dermatomyositis involve:

- Lilac-blue discoloration around the eyelids, cheeks, and forehead, with or without edema.
- Blue-red papules or linear lesions on the dorsum of the hands, elbows, and knees.
- Pigmentation.
- Nail fold telangiectasia.
- Photosensitivity.
- Contractures.

This condition is also associated with malignancy. Further information on dermatomyositis can be found in Chapter 2.

Skin manifestations of systemic disease

Diabetes mellitus

Cutaneous signs of diabetes mellitus include:

- Candidal or bacterial infection—caused by poorly controlled blood sugar levels.
- Ulcers—caused by neuropathy or arteriopathy of the feet.

Systemic features of systemic lupus erythematosus (SLE)	
System	Clinical features
Musculoskeletal	Arthritis
	Tenosynovitis
Cardiovascular	Pericarditis
	Endocarditis
Respiratory	Pneumonitis
	Effusion
	Infarction
Central nervous system	Psychosis
Renal	Glomerulonephritis
Blood	Anemia
	Thrombocytopenia

Fig. 8.23 Systemic features of systemic lupus erythematosus (SLE).

- Eruptive xanthomas—associated with secondary hyperlipidemia.
- Diabetic dermatopathy—pigmented scars on the shins that are associated with diabetic microangiography.
- Necrobiosis lipoidica—yellow-red atrophic plaques seen on shins.
- Granuloma annulare—popular annular lesions found on the hands, feet, and face that fade within a year.

Thyroid disease

Cutaneous signs of thyroid disease are listed in Fig. 8.24.

Cutaneous signs of thyroid disease	
Thyrotoxicosis	**Myxedema**
Skin becomes soft and pink	Alopecia
Hyperhidrosis	Coarse and thickened hair
Alopecia	Skin becomes dry, yellow, and puffy
Pigmentation	Asteatotic eczema
Onycholysis	Xanthomas
Clubbing	
Pretibial myxedema	
Palmar erythema	

Fig. 8.24 Cutaneous signs of thyroid disease.

Hyperlipidemia

Cutaneous signs of hyperlipidemia usually involve xanthomatous deposits. The xanthomas are controlled by treating the underlying hyperlipidemia.

Skin signs of nutritional deficiency and gastrointestinal disease
Malnutrition

Different forms of malnutrition lead to varying skin manifestations (Fig. 8.25).

Inflammatory bowel disease

The skin changes in Crohn's disease and ulcerative colitis vary (Fig. 8.26).

Skin signs of malignancy
Acanthosis nigricans

An uncommon condition associated with malignancy, acanthosis nigricans is characterized by thickening and pigmentation of the skin around the flexures and neck. The skin becomes velvety and papillomatous, and warty lesions develop around the mouth and on the palms and soles. Rarely, the condition may present in childhood; this is an inherited form of the disorder and is not associated with malignancy. When presenting in older patients, a carcinoma, which is most commonly found in the gastrointestinal tract, must be excluded.

Paget's disease of the nipple

A unilateral plaque-like lesion that forms on the nipple areola commonly indicates the spread of an intraductal carcinoma of the breast, called Paget's

Cutaneous signs of malnutrition		
Deficiency	**Disease**	**Cutaneous signs**
Protein	Kwashiorkor	Altered pigmentation Desquamation Ulcers (with brown/red hair in Afro-Caribbeans)
Vitamin C	Scurvy	Purpura Swollen, bleeding gums Indurated (woody) edema
Nicotinic acid	Pellagra	Scaly dermatitis Pigmentation
Iron		Alopecia Koilonychia Pruritus Angular cheilitis

Fig. 8.25 Cutaneous signs of malnutrition.

Skin changes in inflammatory bowel disease	
Inflammatory bowel disease	Cutaneous signs
Crohn's disease	Perianal abscesses Sinuses Fistulae Erythema nodosum Sweet's disease Pyoderma gangrenosum Aphthous stomatitis Glossitis
Ulcerative colitis	Erythema nodosum Sweet's disease Pyoderma gangrenosum

Fig. 8.26 Skin changes in inflammatory bowel disease.

disease of the nipple; an eruption resembling eczema around the perineum or axilla may be caused by intraepidermal malignant spread. With both presentations, a skin biopsy should be performed to confirm the diagnosis.

Erythema gyratum repens
Erythema gyratum repens is an extremely rare disorder that is caused by malignancy, usually of the lung. Scaly concentric rings, which resemble wood-grain and which rapidly change pattern, appear on the body.

Necrolytic migratory erythema
Necrolytic migratory erythema is characterized by serpiginous erythematous plaques that usually begin in the perineum. The eruption is caused by a glucagon-secreting tumor of the pancreas and is associated with weight loss, anemia, diabetes, and angular stomatitis.

Secondary tumor deposits in skin
Skin metastases often present late in malignant disease and therefore carry a poor prognostic value. They usually appear as firm, pink nodules and are found most commonly on the scalp, umbilicus, and trunk. Tumor tissue may metastasize to the skin from the following primary tumors:
- Breast.
- Gastrointestinal tract.
- Ovary.
- Lung.
- Malignant melanomas, lymphomas, and leukemias.

Conditions occasionally associated with malignancy
Other skin conditions that may be associated with malignancy and also with more benign diagnoses include the following:
- Generalized pruritus.
- Acquired ichthyosis.
- Hyperpigmentation.
- Pyoderma gangrenosum.
- Dermatomyositis.
- Erythroderma.
- Hypertrichosis.

A careful history and examination should be obtained from all patients who present with these conditions but who have no obvious underlying cause.

Skin changes in pregnancy
The following skin changes commonly occur in pregnancy:
- Increased pigmentation (especially in the nipples and areolae).
- Chloasma or melasma (mask of pregnancy)—diffuse brownish facial pigmentation.
- Proliferation of melanocytic nevi.
- Development of spider nevi and abdominal striae (stretch marks).
- Pruritus.
- Telogen effluvium (may also occur in the postpartum period).

Drug-induced skin disorders

Most drugs will list an eruption as a side effect, and drug reactions are both common and frequent. Pay attention to a patient who claims to be "allergic" to a drug; although true allergies are uncommon, missing one could lead to dire consequences.

Mechanisms of drug-induced skin disorders
There are several mechanisms that produce a drug-induced skin disorder as shown in Fig. 8.27. The four most important drug reactions are listed in Fig. 8.28.

Mechanisms that produce drug-induced disorders	
Mechanism	**Example**
Excessive therapeutic effect	An overdose of anticoagulants may lead to subcutaneous bleeding and purpura
Pharmacologic side effects	Dry lips and mucosa resulting from use of isotretinoin; bone marrow suppression with use of cytotoxic drugs
Hypersensitivity	True allergy; may occur via any of the four skin type reactions
Skin deposition of drug or metabolites	Gold
Facilitative effect	Use of a drug upsets biologic balance; use of wide-spectrum antibiotics may result in *Candida*
Idiosyncratic reaction	Reaction peculiar to individual

Fig. 8.27 Mechanisms that produce drug-induced disorders.

Important drug reactions				
	Toxic erythema	**Fixed drug eruption**	**Toxic epidermal necrolysis**	**Psoriasiform and bullous eruptions**
Etiology	Caused by drugs (ampicillin, sulfonamides, and carbamazepine), scarlet fever, or viral infection	Quinine, phenolphthalein and sulphonamides often responsible	Drug-induced epidermal necrosis	Lithium and chloroquine exacerbate psoriasis; β-blockers, gold, and methyldopa may precipitate an eruption
Clinical features	Eruption that may be morbilliform or urticarial; may be accompanied by fever or followed by skin peeling; eruption affects trunk more than limbs	Round, redpurple plaques that occur on same site each time drug is taken; lesions may blister and cause pigmentation	Intraepidermal splits in skin: skin red, swollen, and separates as in a scalding injury	Psoriatic eruption
Complications	Recurrence of symptoms drug taken to alleviate	Recurrence of symptoms drug taken to alleviate	Problems in fluid and electrolyte balance; mortality around 25%	Recurrence of symptoms drug taken to alleviate
Management	Stop precipitating drug; clears up within 1–2 weeks	Stop precipitating drug	In-hospital management in intensive care unit	Stop precipitating drug; use emollients if necessary

Fig. 8.28 Important drug reactions.

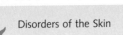
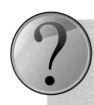

- Differentiate between vesicles, pustules, bullae, and blisters.
- Describe the pathology of dyskeratosis.
- List the five different types of psoriasis, and describe the differences between them.
- Name the topical treatments for eczema.
- Describe the different pathways through which histamine is released in urticaria.
- List the physical features of Reiter's disease.
- Name the condition that sunlight aggravates.
- List the staphylococcal infections that affect the skin.
- Describe the course of an infection with herpes simplex.
- List the factors that predispose an individual to a *Candida albicans* infection.
- Describe the treatments available for scabies.
- Describe the different types of nevi and their distribution.
- Name the risk factors for malignant melanoma.
- List the differences between basal cell carcinoma and squamous cell carcinoma.
- Describe the classification of alopecia.
- List the causes of hirsutism.
- Explain Raynaud's phenomenon.
- Describe the differing pathologies of leg ulcers.
- List the cutaneous forms of malnutrition.
- Name the skin changes in pregnancy.

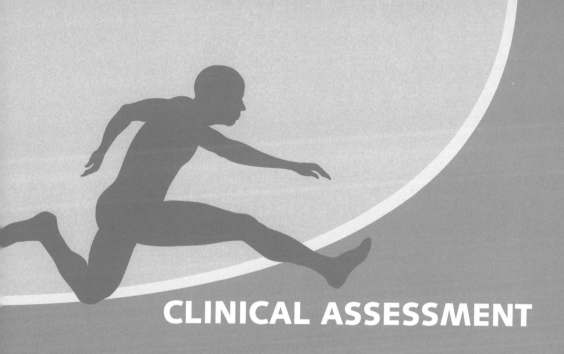

CLINICAL ASSESSMENT

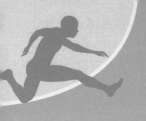

9. Common Presentations of Muscle, Bone, and Skin Diseases

Monoarticular arthritis

Monoarticular arthritis is a common presenting joint complaint (Fig. 9.1). It can be classified into acute and chronic forms.

Acute monoarticular arthritis

Approximately 90% of cases of acute monoarticular arthritis are caused by one of several conditions. These include:
- Sepsis (e.g., from staphylococcal infection).
- Crystal-induced (e.g., gout).
- Trauma.

Chronic monoarticular arthritis

If monoarticular arthritis persists for more than 2 months, it is referred to as chronic (Figs. 9.2 and 9.3).

Polyarticular arthritis

Polyarticular arthritis is inflammation of more than one joint. It can be classified into an acute or chronic form. When the condition lasts for more than 6–8 weeks, it is described as chronic.

Causes of acute polyarthritis include:
- Rheumatoid arthritis.
- Spondyloarthropathies.
- Viral arthritis (e.g., rubella and hepatitis B).
- Systemic lupus erythematosus.
- Acute rheumatic fever.

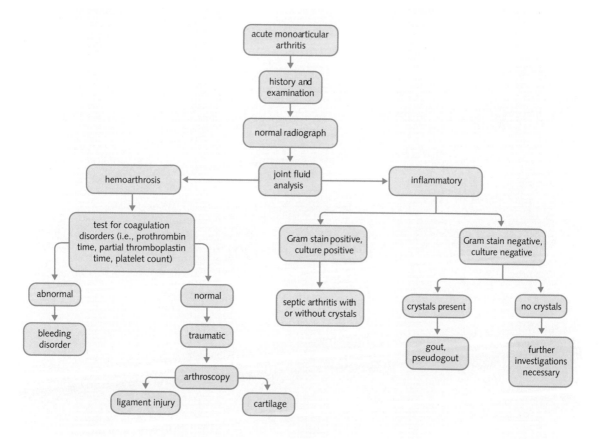

Fig. 9.1 Stages involved in determining a diagnosis of monoarticular arthritis.

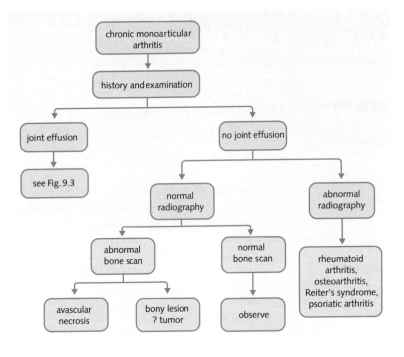

Fig. 9.2 Stages involved in determining a diagnosis of chronic monoarticular arthritis with no joint effusion.

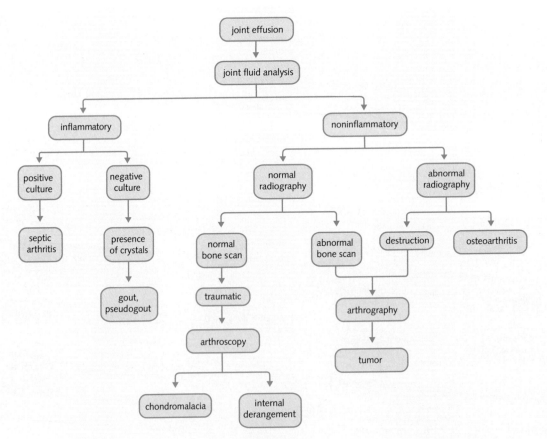

Fig. 9.3 Stages involved in determining a diagnosis of chronic monoarticular arthritis with an associated joint effusion.

Causes of chronic polyarthritis include:
- Osteoarthritis.
- Rheumatoid arthritis.
- Some types of spondyloarthropathies (e.g., psoriatic arthritis, Reiter's syndrome).
- Sarcoid arthritis.
- Systemic lupus erythematosus.

The diagnosis of polyarticular arthritis is aided by a thorough history of the patient because this type of arthritis is often associated with extra-articular features that would indicate the most likely cause (Fig. 9.4).

Back pain

There are four common types of presenting back pain (Fig. 9.5):
- Inflammatory—stiffness after inactivity, with pain relieved by use.
- Mechanical—pain that is aggravated by use and can be associated with symptoms such as locking.

- Neuropathic/referred—pain that is difficult to localize; it may be dermatomal, aggravated by moving the source of the referred pain rather than being attributed to the actual site of pain and may be relieved by rubbing.
- Destructive—progressive pain that may be worse at night; destructive pain usually indicates serious pathology.

1. Inflammatory back pain is caused by:
   - Ankylosing spondylitis.
2. Mechanical back pain is caused by:
   - Acute back strain (damage to either ligaments or muscles).
   - Postural damage.
   - Prolapsed intervertebral disc.
   - Spondylarthritis.
   - Congenital hemivertebrae or sacralization.
   - Fibromyalgia.

Systemic symptoms that may aid diagnosis of polyarthritis		
System	**Symptoms**	**Possible diagnoses**
General	Unexplained weight loss, fatiguability	Systemic lupus erythematosus (SLE), rheumatoid arthritis, ankylosing spondylitis, Reiter's syndrome, sarcoidosis
Eyes	Dryness	Sjögren's syndrome
	Pain	SLE, rheumatoid arthritis, ankylosing spondylitis, Reiter's syndrome, Behçet's syndrome, sarcoidosis
Mucocutaneous	Dry mouth	Sjögren's syndrome
	Rash	SLE, dermatomyositis, psoriasis, Reiter's syndrome, Sjögren's syndrome
	Nail pitting	Psoriasis, Reiter's syndrome
	Subcutaneous nodules	Rheumatoid arthritis, SLE, gout, sarcoidosis
Respiratory	Shortness of breath, pleuritic pain	SLE, rheumatoid arthritis
Gastrointestinal	Symptoms of inflammatory bowel disease	Enteropathic arthritis
Genitourinary	Dysuria	Reiter's syndrome
	Painful intercourse	Sjögren's syndrome, Behçet's syndrome
Musculoskeletal	Muscle weakness	Polymyositis, dermatomyositis, rheumatoid arthritis, SLE, sarcoidosis
	Muscle tenderness, stiffness	Rheumatoid arthritis, SLE
	Joint symptoms	Inflammatory arthritis
Nervous	Headaches and visual problems	SLE

Fig. 9.4 Systemic symptoms that may aid in a diagnosis of polyarthritis.

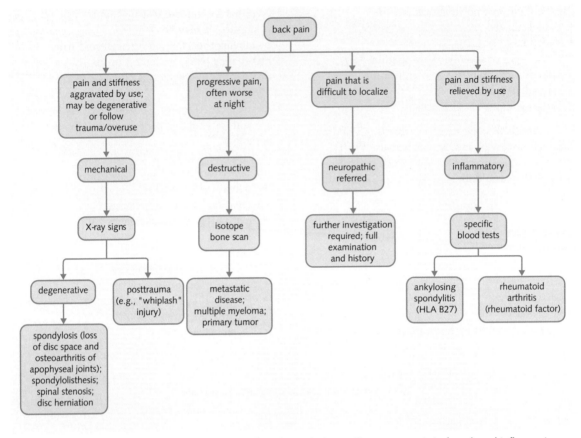

Fig. 9.5 Stages involved in determining diagnoses of mechanical, destructive, neurogenic/referred, and inflammatory back pains.

- Spinal (vertebral canal) stenosis (accompanied by nonreferred pain down into legs).
- Cauda equina syndrome (accompanied by sciatica to below knee).
3. Neuropathic/referred back pain is caused by:
   - Nerve root compression resulting from a prolapsed intervertebral disc; tumor of a vertebra, nerve, or fibro-osseous canal through which the nerve root leaves the spinal column; or spondylosis, abscess, or, less commonly, congenital diastematomyelia and tuberculosis.
   - Referred pain from an intracranial tumor, a pelvic mass, osteoarthritis of the hip, retroperitoneal or urogenital pathology, or aortic dissection.
4. Destructive back pain is caused by:
   - Malignancy.

- Metabolic disturbance (i.e., osteoporosis).
- Sepsis.

Muscle weakness

Patients with muscle weakness can be divided into two categories: those with "true" muscle weakness and those with normal muscle strength.

Muscle weakness may result from disorders occurring anywhere along the motor cortex, corticospinal tracts, anterior horn cells, peripheral nerves, neuromuscular junction, and muscle. (Only the last two of these sites will be considered here.)

Diagnosis of muscle weakness is aided by considering the distribution of the weakness (Fig. 9.6). Further investigations, involving electromyography and muscle biopsy, are

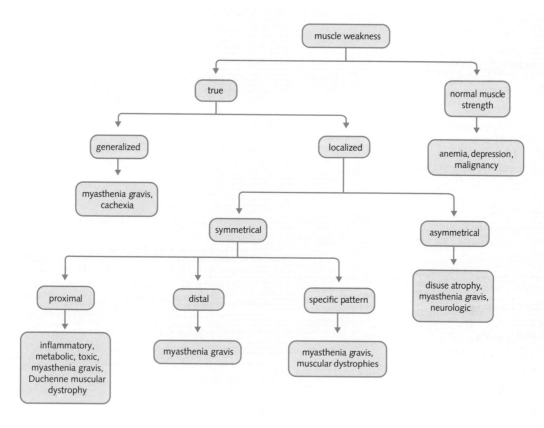

Fig. 9.6 Stages involved in determining a diagnosis of muscle weakness.

required for the definitive diagnosis of muscular weakness.

Common presenting complaints of the skin

Eruptions

Eruptions are generally classified according to their site on the body. They can occur on or in the:

- Face.
- Scalp.
- Feet.
- Hands.
- Anogenital folds.
- Axillae.
- Glans penis.

Facial eruptions are caused by:
- Acne vulgaris.
- Rosacea.
- Atopic dermatitis.
- Contact dermatitis.
- Systemic lupus erythematosus.
- Perioral dermatitis.

Scalp eruptions are caused by:
- Pityriasis capitis.
- Seborrheic dermatitis.
- Psoriasis.
- Tinea capitis.
- Discoid lupus erythematosus.

Eruptions of the hands and feet are caused by:
- Tinea.
- Psoriasis.
- Contact dermatitis.
- Endogenous dermatitis.

Anogenital fold eruptions are caused by:
- Candidosis (in females).
- Tinea (in males).
- Seborrheic dermatitis.
- Psoriasis.

Eruptions in the axillae are caused by:
- Seborrheic dermatitis.
- Psoriasis.
- Contact dermatitis.

Eruptions of the glans penis are caused by:
- Candidosis.
- Psoriasis.
- Lichen planus.
- Scabies.
- Intraepidermal carcinoma.

Blistering

Blistering can occur at several levels of cleavage in the skin. There are common and uncommon causes of blistering.

Common causes of blistering include:
- Friction.
- Insect bites and stings.
- Burns.
- Impetigo.
- Contact dermatitis.
- Drugs.

Uncommon causes of blistering include:
- Pemphigus vulgaris.
- Pemphigus foliaceus.
- Bullous pemphigoid.
- Cicatricial pemphigoid.
- Pemphigoid gestationis.
- Dermatitis herpetiformis.
- Linear IgA disease.

Hypopigmented lesions

Hypopigmented lesions are classified into generalized hypopigmentation and patchy hypopigmentation (with or without inflammation, atrophy, or induration). The causes of generalized hypopigmentation include:
- Phenylketonuria.
- Hypopituitarism.
- Albinism.

The causes of patchy hypopigmentation include:
- Vitiligo.
- Achromic nevus.
- Piebaldism.
- Waardenburg's syndrome.
- Ash-leaf macules.
- Contact with chemicals.

The causes of patchy hypopigmentation with inflammation include:
- Tinea versicolor.
- Leprosy.
- Pityriasis alba.

The common causes of patchy hypopigmentation with atrophy or induration include:
- Radiodermatitis.
- Morphea.
- Lichen sclerosus.
- Burns.

Features that assist in the diagnosis of hypopigmentation can be found in Fig. 9.7.

Hyperpigmented lesions

Hyperpigmented lesions can be split into hyperpigmented nevi and all other causes. A nevus consists of nonfunctional cells and may be defined as a congenitally determined tissue defect.

Hyperpigmented nevi include:
- Congenital melanocytic nevus.
- Acquired melanocytic nevus.
- Mongolian spot.
- Acquired blue nevus.
- Spitz nevus.
- Halo nevus.
- Pigmented hairy epidermal nevus.

The other causes of hyperpigmentation include:
- Tanning.
- Postinflammatory pigmentation.
- Hypoadrenalism.
- Hyperestrogenism.
- Chloasma.
- Metabolic conditions (e.g., cirrhosis, hematochromatosis).
- Chemicals and drugs.
- Freckles.
- *Café-au-lait* macules.
- Peutz-Jeghers syndrome.
- Simple lentigo.
- Actinic (solar) lentigo.

Skin ulcers

Ulcers are skin defects caused by the loss of the entire epidermis and dermis due to trauma, sloughing, or necrosis. They may be venous, arterial, or neuropathic (Fig. 9.8).

Systemic symptoms that may aid in a diagnosis of hypopigmentation	
Cause of hypopigmentation	**Clinical signs**
Vitiligo	Pernicious anemia; Addison's disease; thyroid disease
Albinism	White hair; lack of pigmentation in iris; poor sight; photophobia; nystagmus
Phenylketonuria	If untreated, mental retardation; choreoathetosis

Fig. 9.7 Systemic symptoms that may aid in a diagnosis of hypopigmentation.

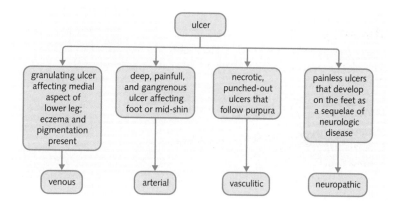

Fig. 9.8 Stages involved in determining a diagnosis of leg ulceration.

Hair loss or gain

Hair loss (or alopecia) can be classified as diffuse, localized, localized scarring, and localized nonscarring (Fig. 9.9). Excess hair is usually termed hirsutism (female with excessive growth of terminal hair in a male pattern) and hypertrichosis (excessive growth of terminal hair in a nonandrogenic pattern) (Fig. 9.10).

Causes of hirsutism are split into five categories:
- Pituitary.
- Adrenal.
- Ovarian.
- Iatrogenic.
- Idiopathic.

Hypertrichosis is classified into localized and generalized.

A

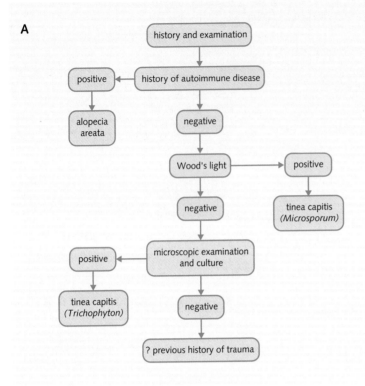

B

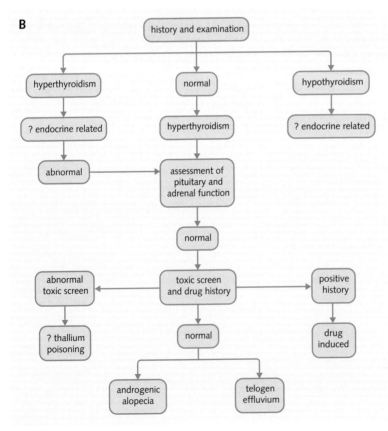

Fig. 9.9 A. Stages involved in determining a diagnosis of localized nonscarring alopecia. B. Stages involved in determining a diagnosis of diffuse nonscarring alopecia.

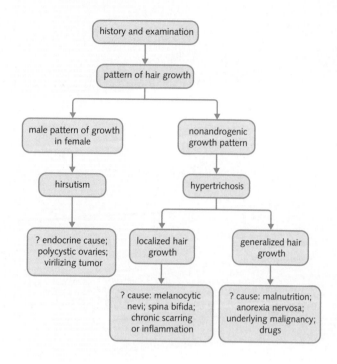

Fig. 9.10 Stages involved in determining a diagnosis of hirsutism or hypertrichosis.

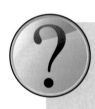

- Name the causes of acute polyarthritis.
- List the four types of back pain.
- Name the causes of anogenital fold skin eruptions.
- What are the common causes of blistering?
- Which nevi are classified as hyperpigmented?

10. History and Examination

Taking a history

Things to remember when taking a history
First contact
When meeting a patient for the first time, you should:
- Always introduce yourself by name and status (e.g., medical student, resident).
- Mention the consultant's or the staff person's name because this reassures the patient that you are genuine and provides a common link.
- Check that the patient is sitting/lying comfortably before you begin.
- Try to put the patient at ease by sitting a reasonable distance away, and take the interview at a relaxed pace; do not worry about any silences between your questions.
- Dress appropriately because many patients feel uncomfortable giving personal details to people who do not look professional—especially if they are scruffy and unshaven. You will obtain better histories if you are suitably dressed.

The patient's surroundings
Try to observe the patient walking into the consulting room; some disabilities can be seen more easily during movement. On the ward, look around the bedside for any clues to the patient's level of disability, or see what the patient brings to the consultation (e.g., an inhaler, oxygen, walking stick/frame, sputum cup, reading material).

The patient's appearance and behavior
Everyone subconsciously makes assumptions about people based on their appearance—you should try to be aware of someone's physical features and clothing.

Watch the patient's behavior for clues while taking the history. For example, is the patient agitated or distressed? Can you see any tremors, abnormal behavior, or abnormal eye and body movements?

Structure of a history for muscles
Presenting complaint
When a patient presents with a muscular complaint, determine the symptoms experienced by the patient (e.g., muscle weakness). These should be recorded in the patient's own words rather than in medical jargon.

History of presenting complaint
Nature of complaint
A patient with proximal weakness (i.e., weakness involving the proximal parts of the arms and legs) will describe difficulties in:
- Getting out of the bath.
- Climbing stairs.
- Getting up and out of chairs.

A patient with weakness of the hands may find it difficult to brush his or her hair. Distal weakness in the limbs is suggested by:
- Difficulties in opening jars.
- Footdrop, in some cases.
- Tripping over rugs.

Patients with myotonia may present with an inability to let go upon shaking hands.

Onset of complaint
The onset of a muscular complaint will depend on the patient's lifestyle. For example, athletes will notice a change in muscle strength at an early stage of a condition. Onset is usually gradual for patients with muscular dystrophies, inflammatory myopathies, and myasthenia gravis. However, the inflammatory myopathies, periodic paralyses, and myasthenia gravis may also present suddenly.

The age of onset is also important. For example, an underlying malignancy should be excluded in older patients presenting with myasthenic symptoms.

Pattern of symptoms
In the case of the inflammatory myopathies and muscular dystrophies, weakness is progressive as opposed to intermittent, as in the periodic paralyses.

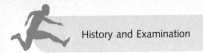

Precipitating or relieving factors

Exercise: An important precipitating factor, particularly in patients with a metabolic myopathy, periodic paralysis, or myasthenia gravis, is exercise. The symptoms of Lambert–Eaton myasthenic syndrome improve with exercise.

Temperature: The myotonia associated with Thomsen's disease and paramyotonia congenita is worse in cold temperatures.

Other associated symptoms

Muscle pain may suggest the viral myalgias (very common), metabolic myopathies, and alcohol excess myopathy. Dysphagia, dysarthria, and respiratory symptoms may be present, depending on the muscle groups involved. Bone pain is suggestive of osteomalacia-induced myopathy.

Past medical history

A history of HIV infection should be excluded for patients with a muscular disorder because the infection itself or its treatment (e.g., administration of zidovudine) may be responsible for myopathy.

Drug history

A range of drugs (e.g., steroids, cholesterol-lowering agents, chloroquine, and lithium) can result in proximal myopathy.

Family history

If other family members are affected by a muscular disorder, a family tree should be constructed. The sex of the patient and affected relatives should be noted.

Social history

Alcohol: When ascertaining the patient's social history, you should ask about alcohol consumption. How much does the patient consume and how often?

Sexual practices: You should try to establish if the patient is at risk of HIV infection.

Exercise: Ask the patient about exercise because the answer to this question can help exclude disuse atrophy.

Review of systems

You should try to establish whether the patient has symptoms of other connective tissue disorders. For example, dark urine is suggestive of myoglobinuria and is associated with metabolic myopathies and acute alcoholic myopathy.

Does the patient have symptoms of endocrine disease, such as Cushing's syndrome or thyroid abnormalities?

Summary of patient's history

Always write a summary of a patient's history when clerking (or interning). When presenting the case, begin with a brief overview of the patient: "Mr. Jones is a 63-year-old man with rheumatoid arthritis who presents with exacerbation of his joint pain." This helps the listener to focus on the relevant parts of the subsequent history.

Structure of a history for joints
Presenting complaint

Presenting complaints of joint disorders are usually:
- Pain.
- Swelling.
- Stiffness.
- Deformity.
- Loss of function.
- Numbness or paresthesia.

History of presenting complaint

For each of the complaints listed in the previous bulleted list, ask when and where the symptom started, if anything makes it better or worse, and how the patient's daily life is affected.

Past medical history

Inquire about any past injuries, because some may predispose the patient to new disorders.

Family history

Genetic disorders should be considered in joint complaints.

Social history

Information about the patient's social life (e.g., occupation and hobbies) can help in a diagnosis.

The "red flags" of musculoskeletal history—those signs that must not be missed—include:
- Pain that wakes the patient up at night.
- Severe, progressive pain that is unremitting.
- Pain accompanied by weight loss.

These signs point to a diagnosis of malignancy or sepsis; both of which must be excluded.

Structure of a history for skin

Presenting complaint

Presenting complaints of skin disorders are usually:
- Rash.
- Itching.
- Psychological distress (e.g., severe acne, extensive psoriasis).

History of presenting complaint

For each of the presenting complaints just described, ask when and where the symptom started, if anything makes it better or worse (e.g., sunlight), and how the patient's daily life is affected. With lesions, ask how and where the problem started, how it first looked, and if it has changed in appearance. Bear in mind that having a skin disease can be very stressful for patients; these patients may frequently devalue their own body image and thus experience psychological distress. However minor the problem may seem to you, it may genuinely cause the patient intense distress and psychosocial impairment.

Past medical history

Inquire about any previous skin disease or atopic syndromes, such as hay fever, asthma, or eczema. Coexisting medical conditions may also involve the skin, and are therefore more relevant.

Drug history

Skin eruptions are one of the common side effects of many prescribed drugs, so take a full drug history.

Also inquire about over-the-counter drugs and alternative medicines (such as herbal remedies) because they may have been used inappropriately and may cause irritant or allergic reactions.

Family history

Skin disorders may be caused by a genetic component (e.g., tuberous sclerosis, psoriasis), but they may also be linked to an infestation or infection that may have affected family members recently. A full family history is therefore important.

Social history

Occupational factors often lead to skin complaints (e.g., chemical engineers with contact dermatitis, health workers with latex allergies). An inquiry into foreign travel may elicit the cause of an infection as well as point toward a reaction to strong sunlight. Taking a sexual history and performing contact tracing may be necessary to determine some disorders (e.g., HIV, syphilis, gonorrhea, vulval disorders).

Communication skills

The dynamics of effective communication

Being able to communicate effectively with patients is one of the most essential skills a clinician can have; after all, the history of a patient makes up 90% of the diagnosis in most cases. Encouraging patients to tell their story, gently dissuading them from irrelevancies, being able to piece together the whole story smoothly, and viewing it in context of the patient's life seems an awesome task at first, but it is one that becomes easier with time and practice.

Communication is a dynamic process and one that is affected by the behavior and character of both doctor and patient. As a medical student, you are faced with handicaps you must understand and deal with before you can establish effective communication with patients, namely:
- The perception that professionals do not show emotions.
- The pressure to feel as if you must be in control of the situation.
- The thought that you must have the answers and therefore be able to act.

- The pressure from peers and tutors to live up to certain expectations.

Identifying and coping with these pressures is the first step in effective communication.

The other factors that affect the doctor–patient dynamic are listed in Fig. 10.1. If they are ignored, a communication gap can ensue. You may think you have imparted appropriate information to the patient, but you may be unaware that the patient has not understood it.

Body language

Traditional images of doctors facing patients across huge desks are now outdated. To put the patient at ease, the doctor must appear and be approachable. If the patient is lying on a bed, sit down to take the history. If the patient is sitting in a chair on the wards, perch yourself on the bed next to the patient. Similarly, if taking a history from a child, bend down to reach the child's level. Do not be afraid to kneel on the floor!

Nonverbal communication

A large proportion of communication between two people does not involve words. The most important components of nonverbal communication are the following:

- Eye contact.
- Facial expression.
- Body language.
- Nonverbal encouragement.

Eye contact

One of the most important tools in communicating is establishing and maintaining eye contact. It plays an important role in establishing trust, obviously an important part of the doctor–patient relationship. Although maintaining eye contact and taking notes is a difficult balancing act, try not to look away from the patient for too long to avoid appearing disinterested.

Facial expression and body language

Most emotion is expressed through facial movements; you can generally tell if a patient is depressed or ecstatic just by looking at his or her face. By studying the patient's facial expression, you can appropriately match your mood to the patient's mood during the consultation. Watch the patient's body language. Is he/she sitting/lying comfortably or squirming and fidgeting? Respond appropriately, and reassure the patient if necessary.

Nonverbal encouragement

Nonverbal encouragement may range from nodding your head while a patient relates his or her story to uttering nonverbal sounds such as "hmmmm" and "uh-huh" during the history. Interaction with patients while they are speaking encourages them to open up and disclose more information.

Verbal communication
Questioning the patient

There is a particular art to choosing which type of question to ask and when to avoid asking at all.

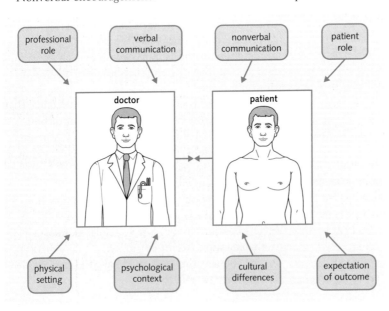

Fig. 10.1 Factors affecting the doctor–patient dynamic.

Questions are classified into open questions, closed questions, and leading questions.

Open questions

Open questions are the best kind to pose when starting a history because they allow the patient to talk. For example, a good open question is "Can you tell me about the pain you have been having?" Listening to the patient's explanation will then lead you into a specific line of questioning. There are times when you need to break in with closed questions, however, to clarify specific points and control the length of the interview.

Closed questions

These questions encourage the patient to give a short (often one-word) answer, and they are helpful in eliciting facts. For example, a closed question may be "Does the pain wake you up at night?"

Leading questions

Leading questions should be avoided because they tend to steer the patient toward an answer. For example, a question to avoid is "I expect this is the worst pain you've ever had?" It is much better to substitute a closed question instead. A better question would be "On a scale of 1 to 10, with 1 being no pain and 10 being the worst pain you have ever had, which number would you assign to the pain?"

Empathizing with the patient

Demonstrating appropriate empathy while taking a history will often encourage patients to disclose information they would not otherwise have stated. Empathy can be expressed simply (e.g., "I understand how hard this must be for you.") or may have a hidden agenda (e.g., "Are you worried that this might be anything in particular?"). Using this approach makes it easy to reassure and relax patients if they have fears and anxieties about their conditions.

Prompting the patient

Although it is better to avoid interrupting while taking a history, sometimes it is appropriate to prompt a patient into a new line of questioning (e.g., "And can you tell me what happened when you got the pain?"). Another way of subtly redirecting the patient's train of thought is to repeat what the patient has already told you (e.g., "So, if I could just recap what you've said . . . .").

Clarifying statements

Do not be afraid to question patients in more detail about their symptoms. If a patient tells you he/she has lumbago, ask him/her if he/she has lower back pain or pain radiating down to the knee. If he/she is having problems with urinating or defecating, ask him/her if he/she is experiencing constipation, urinary incontinence, or perianal numbness.

If you are having problems in assessing your communication skills, ask a patient and staff person for permission to tape yourself taking a history. Listen to the tape and analyze your performance; you may be surprised at how you come across! It is also useful to practice scenarios with friends using timed role play when studying for clinical exams.

General examination of joints and the musculoskeletal system

Clinical examination

It is useful to approach the clinical examination of a patient in a systematic way so that important signs are not missed. All findings should be written down and summarized. You should make sure the patient feels at ease and explain instructions clearly. Remember to look at the patient's face when eliciting signs and to explain your findings at the end of the examination.

When examining limbs, start with either the upper or lower limb, and examine both upper and lower limbs together. It is easier to find an abnormality when there is a normal structure available for comparison. Joints should be examined from the front, back, and sides.

General examination of joints

The routine for examination of joints involves:
- Inspection.
- Palpation.
- Movement.
- Stressing.

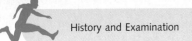

This routine is usually followed by X-rays and imaging studies. It is advisable to examine painful areas last.

Inspection

The area for examination should be adequately exposed and viewed in good light. You should make note of:

- The alignment of the bones—look for any deformities and shortening. Subluxation is present when displaced parts of the joint surfaces remain partially in contact.
- The position of the joint and limbs at rest—is there any unusual posture?
- The joint contour to check for swellings and abnormalities—are there any effusions and general or localized swellings?
- Scars or sinuses—are these from operations (linear scar), injury (irregular scar), or suppurations (broad, adherent, puckered scar)?
- The condition of the skin.
- The presence of muscle wasting.

The terms valgus and varus refer to the deviation of the limb distal to a joint—away from or toward the midline, respectively (see Chapter 2).

Palpation

Palpation includes taking measurements and assessing sensation, movement, and stressing. Preferably with warm hands, palpate gently initially and then more firmly. You should consider:

- Skin temperature changes by noting any warmth (e.g., due to inflammation, rapidly growing tumor) or coldness in local areas.
- Swellings—are they bony abnormalities or diffuse joint swellings?
- Areas of tenderness—these should be precisely located to relate them to anatomic structures.
- Pain—check the patient's face for apprehension during palpation.

Measurements

Measurements of limb length and width are carried out when there are suspected discrepancies between the two sides. Length is especially important in the lower limbs, and width or girth provides information on muscle wasting, soft tissue swellings, or bone thickenings. Refer to fixed points when measuring, and check that the findings are reproducible.

Sensation

An area's sensitivity to light touch and to pinpricks should be assessed. You should precisely locate areas of blunting or loss of sensation.

Movement

Both active and passive ranges of movement must be recorded for the directional planes of each joint. These should be equal: passive movement exceeds active when there is muscle paralysis or torn or slack tendons.

A goniometer, a hinged rod with a scale in the center, is the instrument used for measuring the range of joint movements. Measurements usually begin from the joint positioned in extension, and movement is expressed as degrees of flexion from this point.

The normal ranges of joint movement need to be fully understood, and both sides should be tested. Restricted movements in all directions are suggestive of arthritis, while restrictive movements in some directions and free movements in others suggest a mechanical disorder. Pain and crepitations must also be noted. Joint crepitations are coarse and diffuse, while those of the tendons are fine and limited to the tendon sheath.

Stressing

Straining of the ligaments provides information about joint stability. When assessing ligaments, the muscles moving the joint must be relaxed. If they are contracted, unstable ligaments can be concealed.

Pain is usually present in ligaments that have been recently injured, while those that are torn or stretched produce an increased range of movements. The strength of muscle can be tested by asking the patient to move a joint against the resistance of the examiner. Muscle weakness is easily detectable and a very important sign of motor impairment.

Muscle power is graded as:
- 0: No power.
- 1: A flicker of contraction.
- 2: Slight power to move a joint with gravity eliminated—this is when the joint is supported, usually by the edge of a bed or manually by the observer.
- 3: Sufficient power to move a joint against gravity.
- 4: Power to move a joint against gravity plus added resistance.
- 5: Normal muscle power.

X-rays

Anteroposterior and lateral views of a joint (except for certain joints of the hands and feet) are routinely taken during an X-ray examination. CT and MRI images of bones, joints, and soft tissues are also examined.

Bones

It is important to observe the general outline of bones—are there areas of increased or decreased density? Are there breaks in the continuity of the bone?

Joints

When assessing joints, you should check for:
- Narrowing of the joint space, indicating loss of cartilage thickness.
- Joint margin erosion, typical of rheumatoid arthritis.
- New bone-forming osteophytes, typical of osteoarthritis.
- Flattening or thickening of bone.
- Bone erosion or cavitation.

Soft tissues

In the soft tissues, areas of calcification, foreign bodies, and increased density (suggestive of fluid) should all be noted.

Regional examination of joints and the musculoskeletal system

The principles of general examination are applied to local areas. This section focuses on specific features that should be noted and maneuvers that should be performed.

Examination of the back and vertebral column (spine)
Cervical spine
Inspection

During inspection of the cervical spine, you should note any deformities, such as torticollis, a "cock-robin" posture (lateral flexion caused by cervical erosion from rheumatoid arthritis), and hyperextension (compensation for a small thorax in ankylosing spondylitis).

Palpation

During palpation of the cervical spine, you should check for midline tenderness from a sprain or whiplash injury.

Movement

Movements of the cervical spine include flexion, extension, lateral rotation, and lateral flexion.

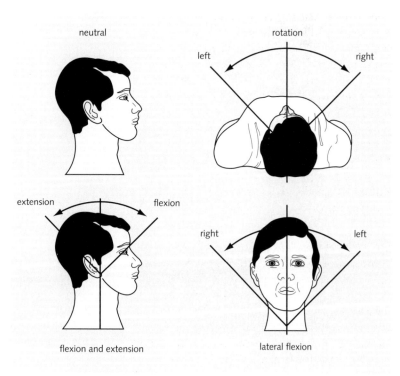

Fig. 10.2 Movements at the cervical spine.

These movements are best seen from the side or front and are expressed as a fraction of the usual range (Fig. 10.2). Restriction of movement occurs in patients with arthritis and nerve compression.

Stressing

Stressing is not useful at the cervical spine.

Thoracic spine
Inspection

During inspection of the thoracic spine, you should note any scoliosis (lateral fixed deviation) or kyphosis (anterior-facing concave curvature); the spine may be rounded or angular due to collapsed vertebrae. This can be achieved by palpating the spinous processes.

Palpation

During palpation, any tenderness of the thoracic spine can be caused by collapse of T12 or L1 vertebrae (e.g., osteoporosis or trauma).

Movement

Movement of the thoracic spine is mainly rotational, but there is a small amount of flexion, extension, and lateral flexion (Fig. 10.3).

Stressing

Stressing is not useful at the thoracic spine.

Lumbosacral spine
Inspection

During inspection of the lumbosacral spine, you should note any lordosis (posterior-facing concave curvature),

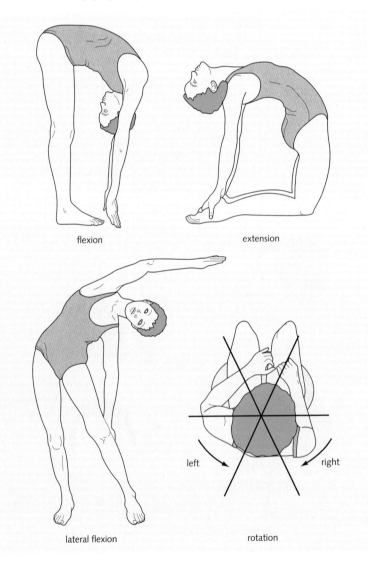

flexion

extension

lateral flexion

left   right

rotation

Fig. 10.3 Movements at the thoracic and lumbar spine.

scoliosis, vestigial ribs on the upper lumbar vertebrae, fusion of L5 with the sacrum (sacralization), and segmentation of S1 (lumbarization). The latter two may require X-ray confirmation.

Palpation

During palpation, any tenderness of the lumbosacral spine may be caused by ligament strain, pain from disc prolapse with vertebral canal narrowing and nerve compression, or perianal anesthesia from a cauda equina lesion.

Movement

Movement of the lumbosacral spine includes flexion, extension, lateral rotation, and lateral flexion (see Fig. 10.3). Restriction follows different patterns (i.e., general restriction in osteoarthritis, asymmetrical flexion in disc prolapse or scoliosis, and painful "catch" on extension in muscle strain).

Stressing

Stressing is not useful at the lumbosacral spine.

Examination of the upper limb
Shoulder
Inspection

During inspection of the shoulder, you should note its contour ("squaring off" in dislocation), swelling caused by effusion (synovitis in subacromial bursa and glenohumeral joint), deltoid muscle wasting, winging of the scapulae (congenital or muscular dystrophies, injury to the long thoracic nerve), alignment of the clavicle and acromion, and the way in which the arms are held (chronic conditions and pain may affect this).

Palpation

During palpation of the shoulder, you may notice that tenderness and pain are localized to different areas in the rotator cuff disorders. This discomfort may be caused by glenohumeral or acromioclavicular arthritis, other arthropathies, or referred pain from other parts of the body.

Movement

Glenohumeral (abduction, adduction, flexion, extension, medial and lateral rotation) and scapular movements (elevation, depression, protraction, retraction, and lateral and medial rotation) (Fig. 10.4) are possible at the shoulder. Circumduction also occurs. You should eliminate scapular movement by pressing the scapula down at the top and asking the patient to move the shoulder. Check the power

of the deltoid (abduct the arm), the serratus anterior (to assess for scapular "winging" when both hands push firmly on a wall), and the pectoralis major (push hands into waist). Check for abnormal movement between the acromion and the clavicle.

Stressing

Stressing is useful at the shoulder when checking for capsular lesions and osteoarthritis.

Elbow
Inspection

During inspection of the elbow, you should look for "gunstock" deformity (malunion of a previous supracondylar fracture), joint effusion swellings, soft posterior lumps (olecranon bursitis), and pebbly osteophytes (osteoarthritis).

Palpation

During palpation of the elbow, you should note any tenderness of the lateral epicondyle ("tennis elbow"), medial epicondyle ("golfer's elbow"), and radial head (rheumatoid arthritis).

Movement

Flexion and extension movements are seen in the humeroulnar joint; supination and pronation can be seen in the radioulnar joints with the elbows flexed at 90 degrees and held into the sides (Fig. 10.5). You should also test the median, radial, and ulnar nerves.

Stressing

Stressing is not useful at the elbow.

Wrist
Inspection

During inspection of the wrist, you should note any deformities or swellings of the tendon sheaths or joint capsule.

Palpation

During palpation of the wrist, you should note any tenderness over the radial area and the anatomic snuff box (e.g., scaphoid fracture, de Quervain's tenosynovitis, osteoarthritis) or the ulnar area (e.g., tenosynovitis of extensors).

Movement

Flexion, extension, adduction (ulnar deviation), and abduction (radial deviation) are the movements at the radiocarpal joint; supination and pronation occur at the superior middle and inferior radioulnar joints (Fig. 10.6).

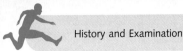

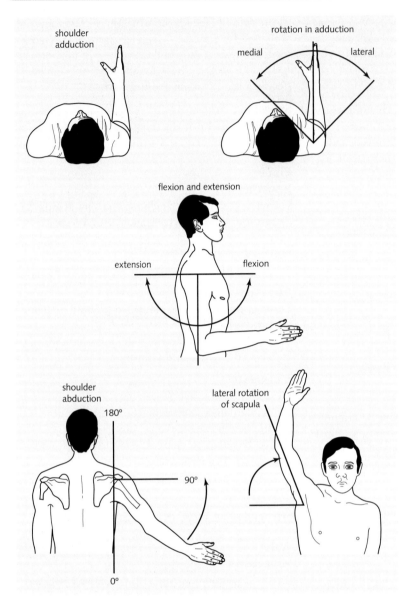

Fig. 10.4 Movements at the shoulder joint.

Stressing

Stressing is not useful at the wrist.

Hands
Inspection

During inspection of the hands, you should look for mallet finger, trigger finger, dropped finger, swan-neck, or boutonnière deformities; a Z deformity of the thumb; ulnar deviation of the fingers (rheumatoid arthritis); Heberden's nodes at the distal interphalangeal joint; Bouchard's nodes at the proximal interphalangeal joints (osteoarthritis); ganglia; and thickening of the palmar aponeurosis (Dupuytren's contracture).

Palpation

During palpation of the hands, you should note any tenderness over the anatomic snuffbox, indicating a fracture of the scaphoid; tender joints occur in patients with rheumatoid arthritis.

Movement

Flexion, extension, adduction, and abduction movements can be seen at the metacarpophalangeal

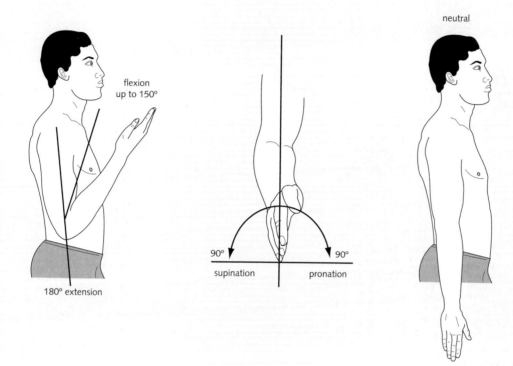

neutral

flexion
up to 150°

90°
supination

90°
pronation

180° extension

Fig. 10.5 Movements at the elbow joint.

joints. There is also opposition of the thumb and little finger (Fig. 10.7). The interphalangeal joints show primarily flexion and extension.

Stressing
Stressing is useful at the hands—applying pressure on the fingers along their axes tests the mechanical stability of the metacarpals and phalanges.

Examination of the lower limb
Hip
Inspection
Inspection of the hip is more useful when it involves watching the gait.

Palpation
During palpation of the hip, you should note any pain at the front of the hip and the skin over the greater trochanter. You should measure the limbs to find their true length (from the anterior superior iliac spine to the medial malleolus, with the angle between the pelvis and limbs equal on both sides) or apparent length (from the xiphisternum to the medial malleolus, with the limbs lying parallel to the trunk).

Movement
Flexion, extension, abduction, adduction, medial rotation and lateral rotation, and circumduction are possible at the hip (Fig. 10.8). You should note any fixed deformities that may be flexed, abducted, or adducted. Fixed flexion can be confirmed by performing Thomas' test. To perform Thomas' test, lay patients down so that they are flat on their back, and place a hand under the lumbar lordosis. Flex the hip and knee of the leg unaffected by fixed flexion; if the other leg also flexes, fixed flexion of the hip on that side

193

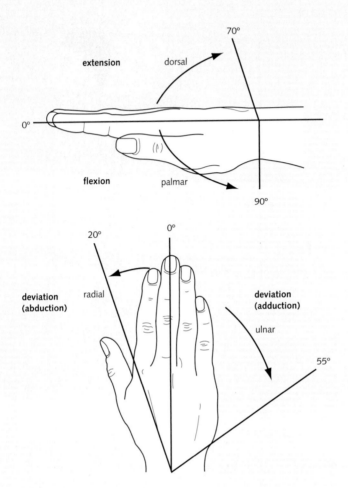

Fig. 10.6 Movements at the wrist joint.

is confirmed, and Thomas' test is positive. Performing a passive leg raise with the knee in extension will allow detection of nerve impingement caused by a slipped disc; it also allows detection of quadriceps lag.

Stressing
Stressing is not useful at the hip.

Knee
Inspection
During inspection of the knee, you should look for genu valgum or genu varum, wasting of quadriceps femoris, and swelling around the knee (thickened bone or synovium, fluid within the joint, or bursitis).

Palpation
During palpation of the knee, you should note any tenderness over the joint due to torn menisci, sprained or torn ligaments, synovitis, or osteoarthritis. Loose bodies may be felt in the suprapatellar region.

Movement
Flexion and extension movements and slight rotational movements are possible at the knee (Fig. 10.9). In some people, the knees can be hyperextended.

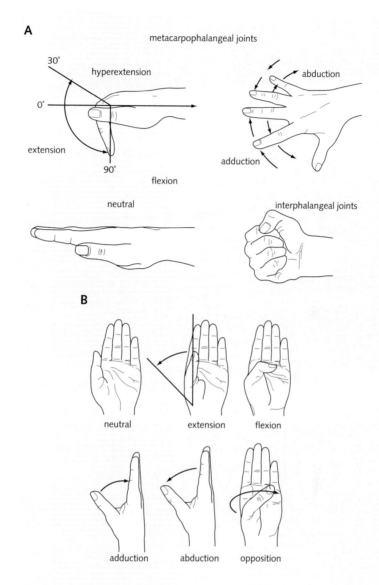

Fig. 10.7 Movements at the finger and thumb joints. A. The finger joint. B. The thumb joint.

Stressing

During stressing of the knee, you should check the collateral ligaments in slight flexion (20–30 degrees) and the cruciate ligaments with the knee flexed at a right angle. These tests are known as the abduction/adduction stress tests and the anterior/posterior drawer signs, respectively.

Ankle
Inspection

During inspection of the ankle, you should check the calf muscles to be alerted to hypertrophic conditions such as Duchenne muscular dystrophy.

Palpation

During palpation of the ankle, you should note any swelling near the joints that may indicate tenosynovitis.

Movement

Plantarflexion and dorsiflexion movements at the ankle are possible (Fig. 10.10). Inversion and eversion occur at the subtalar joint complex.

Stressing

Stressing of the ankle enables checking the integrity of the ligaments.

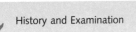
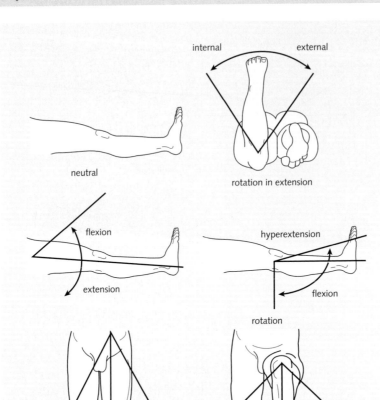

Fig. 10.8 Movements at the hip joint.

Feet
Inspection
During inspection of the feet, you should look for congenital club foot, flat or hollow feet, claw toes, hammer toes, hallux valgus, hallux rigidus, bunions, calluses, and toenail lesions.

Palpation
During palpation of the feet, you should check for a hot and swollen first metatarsophalangeal (MTP) joint. This sign is apparent in patients with osteoarthritis and gout. You should also check the metatarsal heads for prominence and pain.

Movement
Flexion and extension movements occur in the toes; inversion and eversion of the foot occur at the subtalar and midtarsal joints (Fig. 10.11).

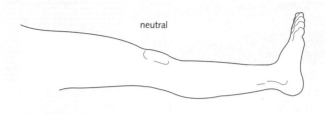

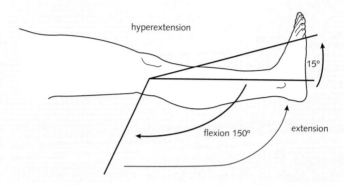

Fig. 10.9 Movements at the knee joint.

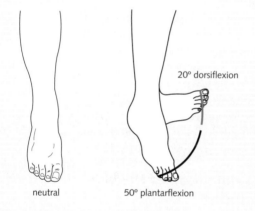

Fig. 10.10 Movements at the ankle joint.

Stressing
During stressing of the feet, you should be able to determine the integrity of the toes by noting the longitudinal pressure.

Examination of the thorax and abdomen
Thorax
Inspection
During inspection of the thorax, you should look for deformities such as pectus carinatum (pigeon chest), pectus excavatum (funnel chest), scoliosis, and "gibbus" (a sharp angular deformity caused by collapsed vertebrae from infection).

Palpation
During palpation of the thorax, you should check for localized tenderness caused by broken ribs or metastasis.

Movement
Any restriction of expansion of the thorax to less than 5 cm is suggestive of ankylosing spondylitis.

Stressing
During stressing of the thorax, you may note that lateral compression causes pain, indicating a broken rib.

Abdomen
Inspection
During inspection of the abdomen, you should look for urethral discharge or balanitis (Reiter's syndrome).

Palpation
During palpation of the abdomen, you should check for splenomegaly (Felty's syndrome),

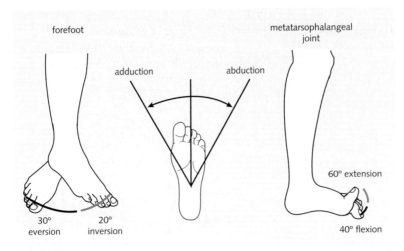

forefoot

adduction   abduction

30°   20°
eversion   inversion

metatarsophalangeal
joint

60° extension

40° flexion

Fig. 10.11 Movements at the foot.

enlarged inguinal lymph nodes (rheumatoid arthritis), and renal enlargement (ankylosing spondylitis).

You should ask the patient about his or her bowel movements. A rectal and stool examination may be useful for the diagnosis of the enteropathic arthropathies, ulcerative colitis, and Crohn's disease.

Examination of the face
Eyes
During examination of the eyes, you should check for any redness and dryness (Sjögren's syndrome), nodular scleritis, and a thin blue sclera (rheumatoid arthritis); cataracts (steroid treatment for musculoskeletal disorders); iritis (ankylosing spondylitis); conjunctivitis (Reiter's syndrome); uveitis (Behçet's syndrome); and difficulty in closing the eyes (scleroderma).

Fundi
At the fundi, look for hyperviscosity (rheumatoid arthritis) or cytoid bodies composed of hard exudates (systemic lupus erythematosus [SLE]).

Mouth
At the mouth, check for dryness and dental caries (Sjögren's syndrome) and ulcers (rheumatoid arthritis, SLE, Reiter's syndrome).

Facies
When examining the facies, you should check for parotid enlargement (Sjögren's syndrome); a cushingoid face (drugs used in rheumatoid arthritis and SLE); an expressionless, pinched "bird-like" face (scleroderma); and alopecia (SLE and scleroderma).

Skin
You should check the skin for butterfly rash (SLE), urticaria and purpura (hypersensitive vasculitis in rheumatoid arthritis and SLE), malar telangiectasia, and skin tethering and pigmentation (scleroderma).

Temporomandibular joint
During inspection of the temporomandibular joint, you should listen for crepitus when the mouth opens or closes (rheumatoid arthritis).

Examination of the skin
Inspection
Ideally, examination of the skin should take place in natural daylight, with full exposure for atypical or widespread lesions. Inspection of the lesions involves noting the distribution and morphology of lesions.

Distribution
Different skin disorders commonly show different patterns of lesion distribution (see Chapter 8). It is important to determine whether the eruptions are symmetrical or asymmetrical, central or peripheral, localized or widespread, and on flexor or extensor surfaces. Some disorders may show specific patterns; for example, shingles erupt in a dermatomal pattern, guttate psoriasis occurs on the trunk, and contact dermatitis usually affects the hands or face.

Morphology

The terminology used to describe skin lesions can be found on pp. 135–137. It is important to note whether the lesions are grouped, linear, or annular and whether they show the Koebner phenomenon.

Skin-derived structures

Examination of the skin should also involve inspection of the hair, scalp, nails, and mucous membranes for associated symptoms.

Palpation

Palpation of skin lesions (a task often feared and hence avoided by medical students) is necessary to assess the constancy, depth, and texture of a lesion. Palpation of lymph nodes is essential in patients with suspected skin malignancy; a full systematic examination is necessary for patients with suspected lymphoma. Peripheral pulses must be assessed in patients with leg ulcers.

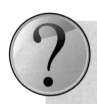

- Name the main points for taking a thorough and effective history of a patient.
- Differentiate between open and closed questions.
- Name the factors involved in the doctor–patient dynamic.
- List three methods of nonverbal communication.
- List the common points of inspection for all joints.
- Describe the normal types and range of movements possible at each joint.
- Explain how to examine the back, shoulders, elbows, hands, hips, knees, and feet for signs of musculoskeletal disorders.
- Describe Thomas' test.
- List the "red flags" that you should note while interviewing a patient about his or her musculoskeletal history.
- Name the areas of palpation in skin examination.

11. Further Investigations

Investigation of musculoskeletal function

Bone densitometry
Density of bone can be estimated by several techniques. These include:
- X-ray computed tomography (CT).
- Magnetic resonance imaging (MRI).
- Radioisotope scanning.

X-ray computed tomography
X-ray CT or computerized axial tomography (CAT) involves X-ray scanning of part of the body from several angles with oscillators that detect the X-rays. Cross-sectional images are then compared and reconstructed by computer. These images can show variation in density between bone and surrounding tissue.

Magnetic resonance imaging
In MRI scanning, the part of the body under investigation is placed in a magnetic field and scanned. Hydrogen nuclei (protons) are lined up in the direction of this magnetic field, assuming a new orientation when the electromagnetic radiation is altered. When the radiation is stopped, the protons return to their original position and emit radiofrequency signals as they do so. These signals can be analyzed and converted into a two-dimensional (2D) image.

MRI scanning can detect variations in density of tissues. It provides a means of scanning without the use of X-rays.

Radioisotope scanning
During routine investigations using radioisotope scanning, an intravenous injection of radiolabeled technetium is administered. Rays emitted from the technetium can be measured with a γ counter or rectilinear scanner.

As the isotope diffuses from bone matrix to blood, its increased uptake provides a measure of hyperemia of bone and increased osteogenic activity.

Electromyography
Electromyography (EMG) is a technique used to record the electrical activity in muscle, both at rest and during contraction.

Method
During EMG, a needle electrode is inserted into muscle. Electrical activity in the muscle is displayed on a cathode ray oscilloscope and heard on a speaker.

EMG is used:
- To determine whether a disorder is caused by disease of the muscle or abnormalities of innervation.
- If there is an abnormality of innervation, which may be localized to the central nervous system, peripheral nerves, or neuromuscular junction.
- To aid in the diagnosis of myopathy, myotonia, and myasthenia.
- To obtain information about the distribution of a disorder so that a biopsy specimen can be taken from the appropriate site.
- To obtain information on the characteristics of motor units.

Assessment of muscle function
Normal muscle
Normal muscle at rest is electrically silent. The insertion of an electrode results in insertional activity because the muscle fibers are mechanically stimulated or damaged. If there is disease, the extent of this spontaneous activity may increase or decrease.

When insertional activity subsides, further activity may be seen only if the electrode is moved or the muscle contracts (Fig. 11.1).

Denervated muscle
Abnormal spontaneous activity of muscle at rest is termed fibrillation potential. However, diseases of the neuromuscular junction and myopathies may also result in this pattern.

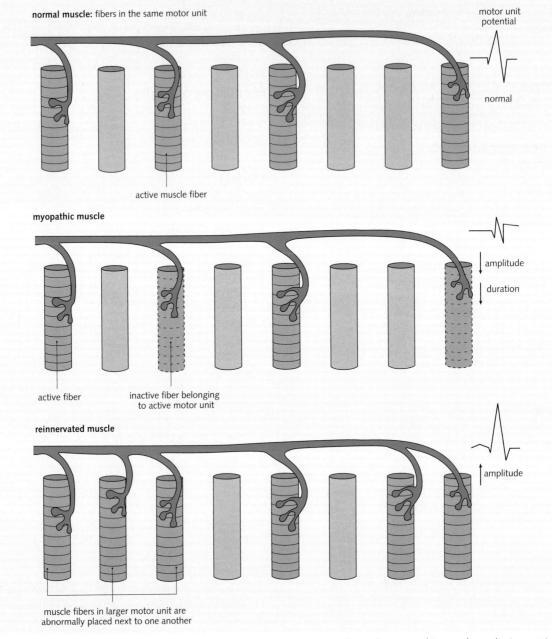

Fig. 11.1 Comparison of the motor unit action potentials recorded in normal muscle, myopathic muscle, and reinnervated muscle.

Myasthenia gravis

Single-fiber EMG is used in the diagnosis of myasthenia gravis. This technique records the time interval between the potentials of two fibers belonging to the same motor unit. In normal muscle, this time interval is 10–50 seconds; in muscle affected by myasthenia gravis, the interval is increased.

Myopathic muscle

In myopathic muscle, the number of active muscle fibers in a motor unit is decreased (see Fig 11.1).

This results in a reduced amplitude and action potential of shorter duration.

Reinnervated muscle

In reinnervated muscle, the muscle fibers are often reinnervated as a result of axonal sprouting of adjacent nerves (see Fig. 11.1). This results in a larger motor unit and, therefore, an increased amplitude of the recorded potential. In addition, there is an unusual arrangement of fibers in the same unit (e.g., they may be rearranged to lie next to each other).

Limitations

EMG does not provide a specific diagnosis because certain types of recording may occur in more than one disorder. It is therefore always important to confirm a diagnosis with clinical findings and laboratory results.

Muscle biopsy
Method

Muscle samples are usually taken by needle biopsy. Local anesthesia is required for this procedure. An open biopsy may be needed to diagnose focal abnormalities, such as myositis.

Evaluation

A muscle biopsy is usually evaluated in one or more ways, including:

- Histology.
- Histochemistry.
- Electron microscopy.
- Assays of enzyme activities.

With these techniques, it is possible to assess muscle fiber types, the presence of inflammation or degeneration, the presence of abnormal mitochondria, and enzyme abnormalities.

Indications

Muscle biopsy differentiates between neuropathic and myopathic disorders. It is used to aid in the diagnosis of a range of inflammatory, dystrophic, and metabolic myopathies.

Investigations of skin disorders

Surgical biopsies

Biopsies are classified as follows: excisional, incisional, punch, shave, or curettage.

Excisional biopsy

Excisional biopsy is not only used to facilitate histologic diagnosis of the lesion, but it is also used to treat the lesion effectively. The lesion is removed along with a defined margin of skin, which depends on the lesion. Biopsies of benign and malignant skin lesions are performed in this manner.

Incisional biopsy

An incisional biopsy is similar to an excisional biopsy, except that less tissue is removed for an incisional biopsy.

Punch biopsy

A punch biopsy is one in which a small (4-mm) punch tool is used to remove a cylindrical section of skin for histologic examination.

Shave biopsy

For a shave biopsy, the lesion is shaved off parallel to the skin surface, with resultant bleeding treated by hemocauterization. This biopsy is only used for benign lesions because some lesion remains; it is usually used for intradermal nevi and seborrheic warts.

Curettage

In a curettage procedure, the lesion is removed using a curette spoon, and bleeding points are cauterized. This method is used to biopsy seborrheic warts, pyogenic granulomas, and viral warts.

Immunologic tests
Prick tests

Prick tests are used to detect immediate (type I) hypersensitivity reactions, and they involve injecting tiny amounts of antigen solutions into the skin of the forearm. After 15 minutes, the skin is inspected, and a wheal of 4 mm or larger is regarded as a positive result. The test is useful for detecting allergies such as those to foods or house dust mites, but it is important that antihistamines are not administered 48 hours before the prick test.

Patch testing

A patch testing procedure detects cell-mediated (type IV) hypersensitivity reactions by applying a standard battery of 23 test substances to aluminum discs that are then taped to the skin. The patches are

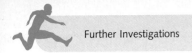

left on for 2 days, after which erythematous patches are correlated to specific test substances. The skin is reexamined after 4 days because some reactions take this long to occur. Patch testing is used in the investigation of contact dermatitis.

Immunofluorescence

Used to diagnose the autoimmune blistering disorders, the immunofluorescence process targets specific immunoglobulins or complement fractions with an antibody labeled with fluorescein (a marker). The marker then shows up under fluorescent light.

An indirect method of immunofluorescence can also be used; this procedure uses animal substrate to reveal certain human serum antibodies tagged with the antihuman immunoglobulin antibody under ultraviolet light.

Wood's lamp

Light from the Wood's lamp emits ultraviolet radiation that causes certain fungal infections to fluoresce on skin and especially hair. It can also be used to detect hypopigmentation, such as that seen in patients with vitiligo.

Microscopy

Skin scrapings treated with a potassium hydroxide solution can be viewed under a light microscope to confirm fungal hyphae. Microscopy is also used in the diagnosis of scabies; the mite can be extracted from its burrow with a needle and viewed.

Routine investigations in musculoskeletal and skin disorders

Hematology
Erythrocyte sedimentation rate

The erythrocyte sedimentation rate (ESR) is the rate at which red blood cells settle out of suspension in blood plasma in anticoagulated blood. A standard ESR tube is used, and the length of clear plasma at the top of the settled blood cells is measured at 1 hour. The normal rate is less than 10 mm/hour. The ESR is raised in inflammatory conditions such as rheumatoid arthritis, systemic lupus erythematosus (SLE), and inflammatory myopathy.

C-reactive protein

C-reactive protein is normally present in small amounts in serum and is synthesized in greater amounts by the liver in response to a variety of insults, including infection. C-reactive protein is raised in inflammatory conditions. It is a more sensitive indicator than ESR, but the results are not available as quickly.

Hemoglobin

Anemia—usually normochromic or normocytic—occurs with inflammatory conditions such as rheumatoid arthritis and SLE.

White blood cell count

The numbers of white blood cells are raised (leukocytosis) in patients with infections, such as septic arthritis.

Thyroid function

The thyroid function test is able to exclude myopathy caused by thyroid dysfunction; parathyroid hormone levels exclude myopathy associated with osteomalacia.

Blood biochemistry
Uric acid

Uric acid levels should be checked if gout is suspected.

Muscle enzymes

Creatine kinase, a muscle enzyme, may be raised in patients with inflammatory myopathy, muscular dystrophy, alcohol myopathy, and metabolic myopathy.

Bone enzymes

Alkaline phosphatase, a bone enzyme, is raised in patients with Paget's disease of the bone, osteomalacia, and rickets, but not in those who have osteoporosis.

Immunopathology
Autoantibodies

Autoantibodies that can be measured in musculoskeletal disorders include:
- Rheumatoid factor in patients with rheumatoid arthritis, Sjögren's syndrome, SLE, polymyositis, dermatomyositis, and sarcoidosis.
- Antinuclear antibodies (ANAs) in patients with SLE (anti-Ro), Sjögren's syndrome, Still's disease, polymyositis (anti-Jo), and dermatomyositis.

	Synovial fluid changes in some rheumatic diseases			
Disease state	Appearance	White blood cells ($\times10^6$/L)	Crystals	Culture
Normal	Clear viscous fluid	<200 mononuclear	None	Sterile
Osteoarthritis	Increased volume; normal viscosity	3000 mononuclear	5% have pyrophosphate	Sterile
Rheumatoid arthritis	May be turbidly yellow or green; low viscosity	30,000 neutrophils	None	Sterile
Septic arthritis	Turbid; low viscosity	50,000–100,000 neutrophils	None	Positive
Gout	Clear; low viscosity	10,000 neutrophils	Needle-shaped; negative birefringence	Sterile
Pyrophosphate arthropathy (pseudogout)	Clear; low viscosity	10,000 neutrophils	Brick-shaped; positive birefringence	Sterile

Fig. 11.2 Synovial fluid changes in some rheumatic diseases.

- Antiacetylcholine receptor antibodies in patients with myasthenia gravis.

Synovial fluid analysis

Synovial fluid should be analyzed for appearance, the presence of white blood cells, and the presence of crystals; the fluid should also be cultured for infections (Fig. 11.2).

Be aware that crystals associated with gout are negatively birefringent, whereas in patients with pseudogout, the crystals are positively birefringent.

Imaging of the musculoskeletal system

The radiograph, or plain X-ray, is the imaging technique most commonly used to diagnose musculoskeletal disorders. It is simple, relatively inexpensive, and quick. However, in some instances, the radiograph may not yield sufficient information; if this is the case, other imaging techniques, such as MRI, CT, or radioisotope imaging, need to be employed.

Normal anatomy

The normal appearance of the musculoskeletal system during imaging is depicted in Figs. 11.3 through 11.10. These include the following:
- Skull (Fig. 11.3).
- Shoulder (Fig. 11.4).
- Elbow (Fig. 11.5).
- Hand (Fig. 11.6).
- Female pelvis (Fig. 11.7).
- Knee and leg (Fig. 11.8).
- Ankle (Fig. 11.9).
- Cervical spine (Fig. 11.10).

Bone disorders
Hereditary disorders
Hereditary bone disorders include the following:
- Congenital scoliosis (Fig. 11.11).
- Osteogenesis imperfecta congenita (Fig. 11.12).

Infections and trauma
Bone is prone to infection, called osteomyelitis (Fig. 11.13), and trauma.

Metabolic disease
Metabolic bone disorders include the following:
- Hyperparathyroidism (Fig. 11.14).
- Vitamin D deficiency (Fig. 11.15).
- Periarticular osteoporosis (Fig. 11.16).

Tumors
Hereditary bone tumors include the following:
- Osteosarcoma (Fig. 11.17).
- Giant-cell tumor (Fig. 11.18).

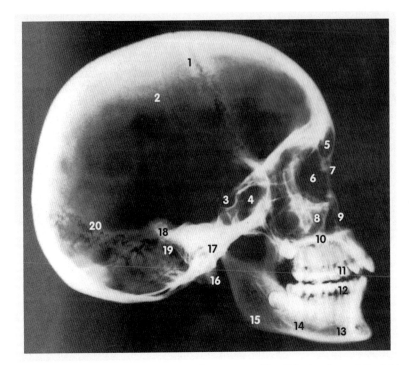

1. Coronal suture.
2. Grooves for meningeal vessels.
3. Pituitary fossa.
4. Sphenoidal sinus.
5. Frontal sinus.
6. Orbit.
7. Nasal bones.
8. Maxillary sinus.
9. Anterior nasal spine.
10. Hard palate.
11. Maxilla and teeth.
12. Mandible and teeth.
13. Mental foramen.
14. Mandibular canal.
15. Angle of mandible.
16. Mastoid process.
17. External acoustic meatus.
18. Petrous ridge.
19. Groove for sigmoid sinus.
20. Lambdoid suture.

Fig. 11.3 Lateral radiograph of the skull (courtesy of Dr. B Berkovitz and Dr. B Moxham).

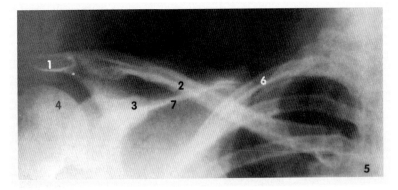

1. Acromion process of scapula.
2. Clavicle.
3. Coracoid process of scapula.
4. Head of humerus.
5. Manubrium.
6. Ribs.
7. Spine of scapula.

Fig. 11.4 Radiograph of the right shoulder (courtesy of Dr. J Calder and Dr. G Chessell).

206

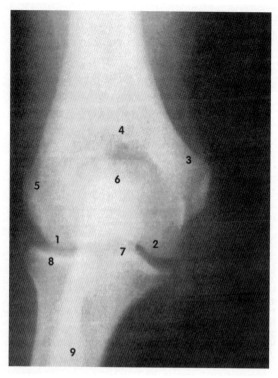

1. Capitulum of humerus.
2. Trochlea of humerus.
3. Medial epicondyle of humerus.
4. Olecranon fossa of humerus.
5. Lateral epicondyle of humerus.
6. Olecranon process of ulna.
7. Coronoid process of ulna.
8. Head of radius.
9. Radial tuberosity.

Fig. 11.5 Anteroposterior radiograph of the right elbow (courtesy of Dr. J Calder and Dr. G Chessell).

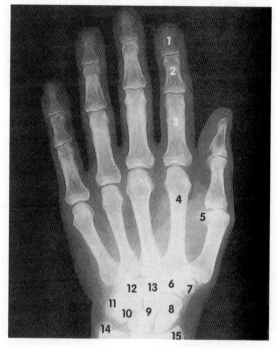

1. Distal phalanx.
2. Middle phalanx.
3. Proximal phalanx.
4. Second metacarpal.
5. Sesamoid bone.
6. Trapezoid.
7. Trapezium.
8. Scaphoid.
9. Lunate.
10. Triquetrum.
11. Pisiform.
12. Hamate.
13. Capitate.
14. Styloid process of ulna.
15. Styloid process of radius.

Fig. 11.6 Radiograph of an adult hand (courtesy of Dr. J Gosling, Dr. P Harris, Dr. J Humpherson, Dr. I Whitmore, and Dr. P Willan).

1. Iliac crest.
2. Anterior superior iliac spine.
3. Anterior inferior iliac spine.
4. Pelvic brim.
5. Sacroiliac joint.
6. Superior pubic ramus.
7. Obturator foramen.
8. Inferior ischial ramus.
9. Inferior pubic ramus.
10. Body of pubis.
11. Pubic symphysis.
12. Subpubic arch.
13. Acetabulum.
14. Head of femur.
15. Neck of femur.
16. Greater trochanter of femur.
17. Lesser trochanter of femur.

Fig. 11.7 Anteroposterior radiograph of the female pelvis (courtesy of Dr. J Calder and Dr. G Chessell).

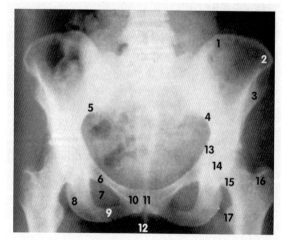

207

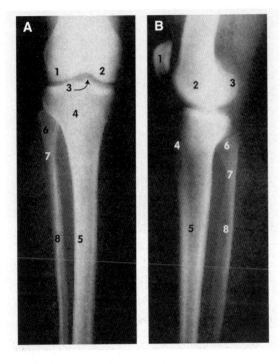

A
1. Lateral femoral condyle.
2. Medial femoral condyle.
3. Tibial spine.
4. Tibial tuberosity.
5. Shaft of tibia.
6. Head of fibula.
7. Neck of fibula.
8. Shaft of fibula.

B
1. Patella.
2. Medial femoral condyle.
3. Lateral femoral condyle.
4. Tibial tuberosity.
5. Shaft of tibia.
6. Head of fibula.
7. Neck of fibula.
8. Shaft of fibula.

Fig. 11.8 Radiographs of the knee and leg.
A. Anteroposterior radiograph of the right tibia and fibula.
B. Lateral radiograph of the right tibia and fibula (courtesy of Dr. J Calder and Dr. G Chessell).

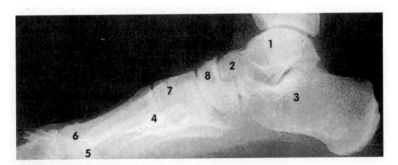

1. Medial malleolus.
2. Head of talus.
3. Calcaneus.
4. Base of first metatarsal.
5. Sesamoid bone.
6. Head of first metatarsal.
7. Cuneiforms.
8. Navicular.

Fig. 11.9 Radiograph of the right foot and ankle showing longitudinal arches (courtesy of Dr. J Gosling, Dr. P Harris, Dr. J Humpherson, Dr. I Whitmore, and Dr. P Willan).

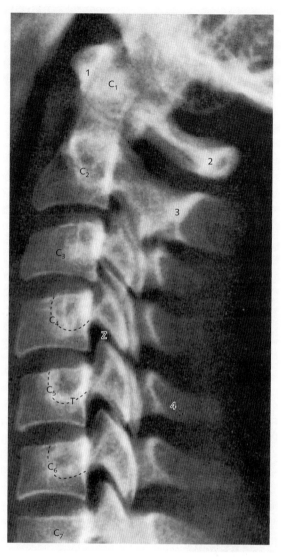

1. Anterior arch of atlas (C_1).
2. Posterior arch of atlas (C_1).
3. Spinous process of axis (C_2).
4. Spinous process of C_5.
C_1–C_7. Bodies of cervical vertebrae.
Z. Facet or zygaphophyseal joint.
T. Transverse process.
Fig. 11.10 Lateral radiograph of the cervical spine (courtesy of Dr. A Greenspan and Dr. P Montesano).

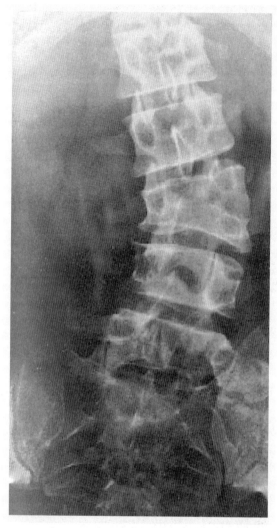

Fig. 11.11 Congenital scoliosis. This case of scoliosis in a 22-year-old man was due to hemivertebrae—a complete unilateral failure of formation (courtesy of Dr. A Greenspan).

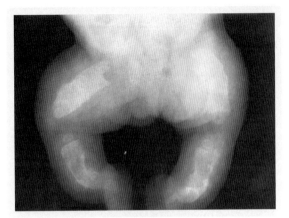

Fig. 11.12 Osteogenesis imperfecta congenita. This infant was born with type II osteogenesis imperfecta, characterized by multiple fractures present before birth. The patient has gross deformity of the lower limbs with multiple healing fractures (courtesy of Dr. T Lissauer).

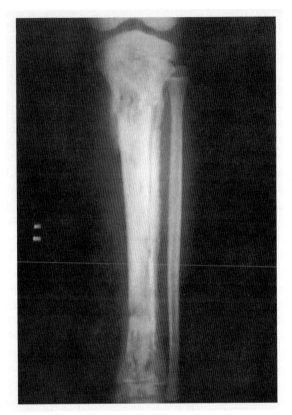

Fig. 11.13 Osteomyelitis. This chronic case shows a periosteal reaction along the lateral shaft of the tibia and multiple hypodense areas in the metaphyseal region (courtesy of Dr. T Lissauer).

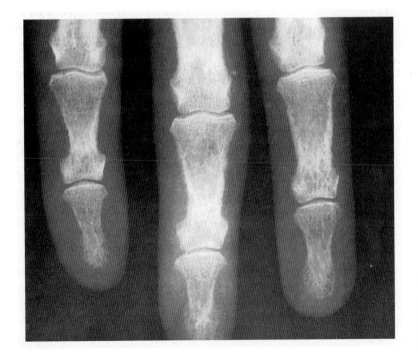

Fig. 11.14 Hyperparathyroidism. The terminal phalanges show tufting and subperiosteal lesions, characteristic signs of primary hyperparathyroidism (courtesy of Dr. PM Bouloux).

A

B

C

D

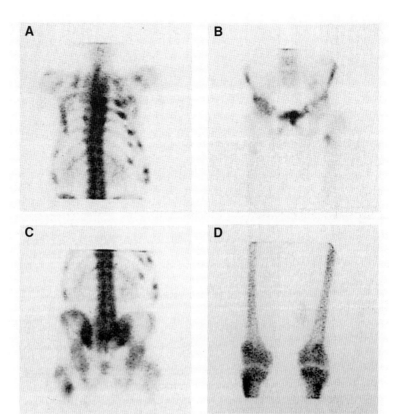

Fig. 11.15 Radioisotope bone scan showing a generalized increase in technetium uptake with multiple hot spots due to small fractures. The patient had metabolic bone disease caused by vitamin D deficiency. The darker areas indicate increased uptake of technetium, representing altered cell growth. A. Thoracic spine. B. Pelvis. C. Lumbar spine. D. Femur and knee joint (courtesy of Dr. PM Bouloux).

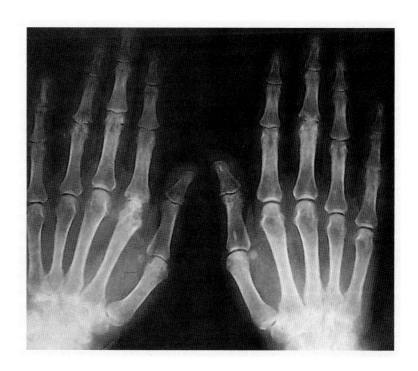

Fig. 11.16 Periarticular osteoporosis with mild ulnar changes in early rheumatoid arthritis (courtesy of Dr. PM Bouloux).

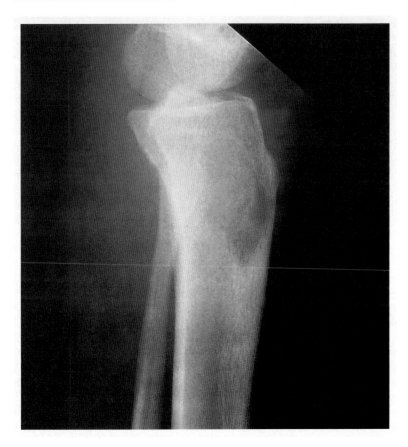

Fig. 11.17 Osteosarcoma in a child. The radiograph shows an infiltrative, poorly demarcated tumor in the metaphyseal region of the tibia (courtesy of Dr. S Taylor).

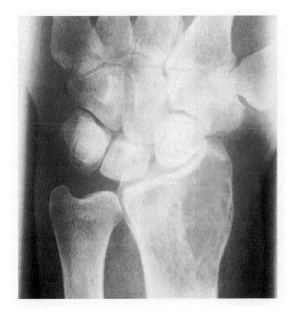

Fig. 11.18 Giant-cell tumor of the radius. Radiograph of the left wrist shows an expanding lytic lesion replacing the distal radius. The lesion is epiphyseal and abuts the adjacent articular surface. There is thinning of the radial cortex but no periosteal reaction and no reactive sclerosis at the proximal extent of the lesion (courtesy of Mr. WA Jones).

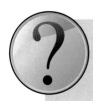

- List the techniques available to determine bone density.
- Explain the uses and limitations of the EMG technique.
- Describe the technique of muscle biopsy.
- List the important blood tests in investigating the musculoskeletal system.
- Describe the characteristics of synovial fluid found in patients with osteoarthritis, rheumatoid arthritis, and septic arthritis.
- Explain three ways of measuring bone density.
- Identify the diseases with which rheumatoid factor is associated and detected.
- List some methods of assessing muscle function.
- List routine laboratory investigations to assess musculoskeletal function.
- Interpret normal radiographs of the skeleton.
- Spot abnormalities in radiographs of diseased skeletons.
- Name the skin disorders that can be diagnosed by the use of a light microscope.
- Differentiate between prick tests and spot tests.
- List the techniques used for biopsy of the skin.
- Explain when it is necessary to use a Wood's lamp.

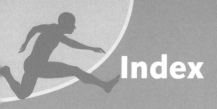

Index

Page numbers for figures are indicated by bold type.

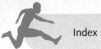

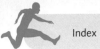

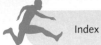

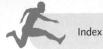

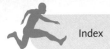

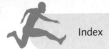

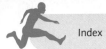

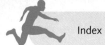